EYE, BRAIN, AND VISION

David H. Hubel

SCIENTIFIC
AMERICAN
LIBRARY

A division of HPHLP
New York

Library of Congress Cataloging-in-Publication Data

Hubel, David H.
  Eye, brain, and vision.

  (Scientific American Library series; #22)
  Bibliography: p.
  Includes index.
  1. Visual cortex. 2. Vision. I. Title.
II. Series: Scientific American Library series;
no. 22 [DNLM: 1. Eye—physiology. 2. Vision—
physiology. 3. Visual Cortex—physiology. WW 103 H877e]
QP383.H83   1987   612'.84   87-23506
ISBN 0-7167-5020-1
ISBN 0-7167-6009-6 (pbk)

Printed in the United States of America

Scientific American Library
A division of HPHLP
New York

Distributed by W. H. Freeman and Company
41 Madison Avenue, New York, New York 10010 and
20 Beaumont Street, Oxford OX1 2NQ, England

1 2 3 4 5 6 7 8 9 0   KP   9 9 8 7 6 5

This book is number 22 of a series.

CONTENTS

PREFACE

This book is mainly about the development of our ideas on how the brain handles visual information; it covers roughly the period between 1950 and 1980. The book is unabashedly concerned largely with research that I have been involved in or have taken a close interest in. I count myself lucky to have been around in that era, a time of excitement and fun. Some of the experiments have been arduous, or so it has often seemed at 4:00 A.M., especially when everything has gone wrong. But 98 percent of the time the work is exhilarating. There is a special immediacy to neurophysiological experiments: we can see and hear a cell respond to the stimuli we use and often realize, right at the time, what the responses imply for brain function. And in modern science, neurobiology is still an area in which one can work alone or with one colleague, on a budget that is minuscule by the standards of particle physics or astronomy.

To have trained and worked on the North American continent has been a special piece of good luck, given the combination of a wonderful university system and a government that has consistently backed research in biology, especially in vision. I can only hope that we have the sense to cherish and preserve such blessings.

In writing the book I have had the astronomer in mind as my prototypical reader—someone with scientific training but not an expert in biology, let alone neurobiology. I have tried to give just enough background to make the neurobiology comprehensible, without loading the text down with material of interest only to experts. To steer a course between excessive superficiality and excessive detail has not been easy, especially because the very nature of the brain compels us to look at a wealth of articulated, interrelated details in order to come away with some sense of what it is and does.

All the research described here, in which I have played any part, has been the outcome of joint efforts. From 1958 to the late 1970s my work was in partnership with Torsten Wiesel. Had it not been for his ideas, energy, enthusiasm,

stamina, and willingness to put up with an exasperating colleague, the outcome would have been very different. Both of us owe a profound debt to
Stephen Kuffler, who in the early years guided our work with the lightest
hand imaginable, encouraged us with his boundless enthusiasm, and occasionally discouraged our duller efforts simply by looking puzzled.

For help in writing one needs critics (*I* certainly do)—the harsher and more
unmerciful, the better. I owe a special debt to Eric Kandel for his help with the
emphasis in the opening three chapters, and to my colleague Margaret Livingstone, who literally tore three of the chapters apart. One of her comments
began, "First you are vague, and then you are snide . . . ." She also tolerated
much irascibility and postponement of research. To the editors of the Scientific American Library, notably Susan Moran, Linda Davis, Gerard Piel, and
Linda Chaput, and to the copyeditor, Cynthia Farden, I owe a similar debt: I
had not realized how much a book depends on able and devoted editors. They
corrected countless English solecisms, but their help went far beyond that, to
spotting duplications, improving clarity, and tolerating my insistence on placing commas and periods after quotation marks. Above all, they would not
stop bugging me until I had written the ideas in an easily understandable (I
hope!) form. I want to thank Carol Donner for her artwork, as well as Nancy
Field, the designer, Melanie Nielson, the illustration coordinator, and Susan
Stetzer, the production coordinator. I am also grateful for help in the form of
critical reading from Susan Abookire, David Cardozo, Whittemore Tingley,
Deborah Gordon, Richard Masland, and Laura Regan. As always, my secre-
tary, Olivia Brum, was helpful to the point of being indispensable and tolerant
of my moods beyond any reasonable call of duty. My wife, Ruth, contributed
much advice and put up with many lost weekends. It will be a relief not to
have to hear my children say, "Daddy, when are you going to finish that
book?" It has, at times, seemed as remote a quest as Sancho Panza's island.

David H. Hubel

The changes I have made for this paperback edition consist mainly of minor
corrections, the most embarrassing of which is the formula for converting
degrees to radians. My high school mathematics teachers must be turning over
in their graves. I have not made any attempt to incorporate recent research on
the visual cortex, which in the last ten years has mostly focussed on areas
beyond the striate cortex. To extend the coverage to include these areas would
have required another book. I did feel that it would be unforgivable not to say
something about two major advances: the work of Jeremy Nathans on the
genetics of visual pigments, and recent work on the development of the visual
system, by Carla Schatz, Michael Stryker, and others.

David H. Hubel
January 1995

Eye, Brain, and Vision

Santiago Ramón y Cajal playing chess (white) in 1898, at an age of about 46, while on vacation in Miraflores de la Sierra. This picture was taken by one of his children. Most neuroanatomists would agree that Ramón y Cajal stands out far before anyone else in their field and probably in the entire field of central-nervous neurobiology. His two major contributions were (1) establishing beyond reasonable doubt that nerve cells act as independent units, and (2) using the Golgi method to map large parts of the brain and spinal cord, so demonstrating both the extreme complexity and extreme orderliness of the nervous system. For his work he, together with Golgi, received the Nobel Prize in 1906.

1

INTRODUCTION

Intuition tells us that the brain is complicated. We do complicated things, in immense variety. We breathe, cough, sneeze, vomit, mate, swallow, and urinate; we add and subtract, speak, and even argue, write, sing, and compose quartets, poems, novels, and plays; we play baseball and musical instruments. We perceive and think. How could the organ responsible for doing all that not be complex?

We would expect an organ with such abilities to have a complex structure. At the very least, we would expect it to be made up of a large number of elements. That alone, however, is not enough to guarantee complexity. The brain contains 10^{12} (one million million) cells, an astronomical number by any standard. I do not know whether anyone has ever counted the cells in a human liver, but I would be surprised if it had fewer cells than our brain. Yet no one has ever argued that a liver is as complicated as a brain.

We can see better evidence for the brain's complexity in the interconnections between its cells. A typical nerve cell in the brain receives information from hundreds or thousands of other nerve cells and in turn transmits information to hundreds or thousands of other cells. The total number of interconnections in the brain should therefore be somewhere around 10^{14} to 10^{15}, a larger number, to be sure, but still not a reliable index of complexity. Anatomical complexity is a matter not just of numbers; more important is intricacy of organization, something that is hard to quantify. One can draw analogies between the brain and a gigantic pipe organ, printing press, telephone exchange, or large computer, but the usefulness of doing so is mainly in conveying the image of a large number of small parts arranged in precise order, whose functions, separately or together, the nonexpert does not grasp. In fact, such analogies work best if we happen not to have any idea how printing presses and telephone exchanges work. In the end, to get a feeling for what the brain is and how it is organized and handles information, there is no substitute for examining it, or parts of it, in detail. My hope in this book is to convey some flavor of the brain's structure and function by taking a close look at the part of it concerned with vision.

The questions that I will be addressing can be simply stated. When we look at the outside world, the primary event is that light is focused on an array of 125 million receptors in the retina of each eye. The receptors, called *rods* and *cones,* are nerve cells specialized to emit electrical signals when light hits them. The task of the rest of the retina and of the brain proper is to make sense of these signals, to extract information that is biologically useful to us. The result is the scene as we perceive it, with all its intricacy of form, depth, movement, color, and texture. We want to know how the brain accomplishes this feat.

Before I get your hopes and expectations too high I should warn you that we know only a small part of the answer. We do know a lot about the machinery of the visual system, and we have a fair idea how the brain sets about the task. What we know is enough to convince anyone that the brain, though complicated, works in a way that will probably someday be understood—and that the answers will not be so complicated that they can be understood only by people with degrees in computer science or particle physics.

Today we have a fairly satisfactory understanding of most organs of our body. We know reasonably well the functions of our bones, our digestive tubes, our kidneys and liver. Not that everything is known about any of these—but at least we have rough ideas: that digestive tubes deal with food, the heart pumps blood, bones support us, and some bones make blood. (It would be hard to imagine a time, even in the dark twelfth century, when it was not appreciated that bones are what make our consistency different from that of an earthworm, but we can easily forget that it took a genius like William Harvey to discover what the heart does.) What something is *for* is a question that applies only to biology, in the broad sense of the word "biology." We can ask meaningfully what a rib is for: it supports the chest and keeps it hollow. We can ask what a bridge is for: it lets humans cross a river— and humans, which are part of biology, invented the bridge. Purpose has no meaning outside of biology, so that I laugh when my son asks me, "Daddy, what's snow for?" How purpose comes into biology has to do with evolution, survival, sociobiology, selfish genes—any number of exalted topics that keep many people busy full time. Most things in anatomy—to return to solid ground—even such erstwhile mysterious structures as the thymus gland and the spleen, can now have quite reasonable functions assigned to them. When I was a medical student, the thymus and spleen were question marks.

The brain is different. Even today large parts of it are question marks, not only in terms of how they work but also in terms of their biological purpose. A huge, rich subject, neuroanatomy consists largely of a sort of geography of

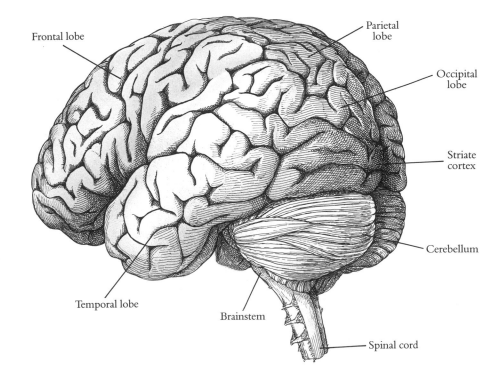

Frontal lobe

Parietal
lobe

Occipital
lobe

Striate
cortex

Cerebellum

Temporal lobe

Brainstem

Spinal cord

This view of a human brain seen from the
left and slightly behind shows the cerebral
cortex and cerebellum. A small part of the
brainstem can be seen just in front of the
cerebellum.

structures, whose functions are still a partial or complete mystery. Our ignorance of these regions is of course graded. For example, we know a fair
amount about the region of brain called the motor cortex and have a rough
idea of its function: it subserves voluntary movement; destroy it on one side
and the hand and face and leg on the opposite side become clumsy and weak.
Our knowledge of the motor cortex lies midway along a continuum of relative knowledge that ranges all the way from utter ignorance of the functions of
some brain structures to incisive understanding of a few—like the understanding we have of the functions of a computer, printing press, internal combus-
tion engine, or anything else we invented ourselves.

The visual pathway, in particular the *primary visual cortex*, or *striate cortex*,
lies near the bone or heart end of this continuum. The visual cortex is perhaps
the best-understood part of the brain today and is certainly the best-known
part of the cerebral cortex. We know reasonably well what it is "for", which is
to say that we know what its nerve cells are doing most of the time in a
person's everyday life and roughly what it contributes to the analysis of the

visual information. This state of knowledge is quite recent, and I can well remember, in the 1950s, looking at a microscopic slide of visual cortex, showing the millions of cells packed like eggs in a crate, and wondering what they all could conceivably be doing, and whether one would ever be able to find out.

How should we set about finding out? Our first thought might be that a detailed understanding of the connections, from the eye to the brain and within the brain, should be enough to allow us to deduce how it works. Unfortunately, that is only true to a limited extent. The regions of cortex at the back of the human brain were long known to be important for vision partly because around the turn of the century the eyes were discovered to make connections, through an intermediate way station, to this part of the brain. But to deduce from the structure alone what the cells in the visual cortex are doing when an animal or person looks at the sky or a tree would require a knowledge of anatomy far exceeding what we possess even now. And we would have trouble even if we did have a complete circuit diagram, just as we would if we tried to understand a computer or radar set from their circuit diagrams alone—especially if we did not know what the computer or radar set was for.

Our increasing knowledge of the working of the visual cortex has come from a combination of strategies. Even in the late 1950s, the physiological method of recording from single cells was starting to tell us roughly what the cells were doing in the daily life of an animal, at a time when little progress was being made in the detailed wiring diagram. In the past few decades both fields, physiology and anatomy, have gone ahead in parallel, each borrowing techniques and using new information from the other.

I have sometimes heard it said that the nervous system consists of huge numbers of random connections. Although its orderliness is indeed not always obvious, I nevertheless suspect that those who speak of random networks in the nervous system are not constrained by any previous exposure to neuroanatomy. Even a glance at a book such as Cajal's *Histologie du Système Nerveux* should be enough to convince anyone that the enormous complexity of the nervous system is almost always accompanied by a compelling degree of orderliness. When we look at the orderly arrays of cells in the brain, the impression is the same as when we look at a telephone exchange, a printing press, or the inside of a TV set—that the orderliness surely serves some purpose. When confronted with a human invention, we have little doubt that the whole machine and its separate parts have understandable functions. To understand them we need only read a set of instructions. In biology we develop a similar faith in the functional validity and even ultimately in the understandability of structures that were not invented, but were perfected through millions of years of evolution. The problem of the neurobiologist (to be sure, not the only problem) is to learn how the order and complexity relate to the function.

To begin, I want to give you a simplified view of what the nervous system is like—how it is built up, the way it works, and how we go about studying it. I will describe typical nerve cells and the structures that are built from them.

The main building blocks of the brain are the nerve cells. They are not the only cells in the nervous system: a list of all the elements that make up the brain would also include glial cells, which hold it together and probably also help nourish it and remove waste products; blood vessels and the cells that they are made of; various membranes that cover the brain; and I suppose even the skull, which houses and protects it. Here I will discuss only the nerve cells.

Many people think of nerves as analogous to thin, threadlike wires along which electrical signals run. But the nerve fiber is only one of many parts of the nerve cell, or *neuron*. The *cell body* has the usual globular shape we associate with most cells (see diagram on this page) and contains a nucleus, mitochondria, and the other organelles that take care of the many housekeeping functions that cell biologists love to talk about. From the cell body comes the main cylinder-shaped, signal-transmitting nerve fiber, called the *axon*. Besides the axon, a number of other branching and tapering fibers come off the cell body:

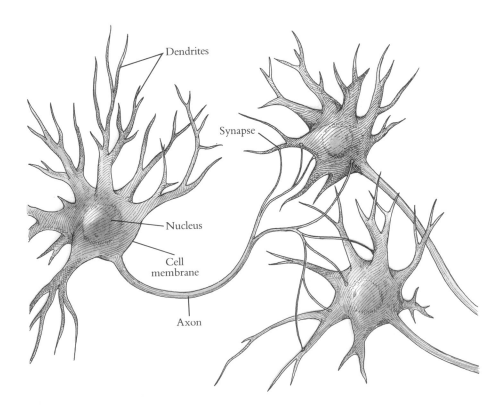

Dendrites

Synapse

Nucleus

Cell membrane

Axon

The principal parts of the nerve cell are the cell body containing the nucleus and other organelles; the single axon, which conveys impulses from the cell; and the dendrites, which receive impulses from other cells.

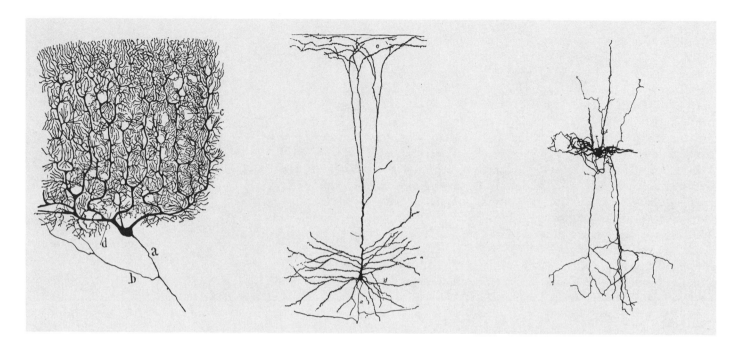

Left: The cerebellar Purkinje cell, shown in a drawing by Santiago Ramón y Cajal, presents an extreme in neuronal specialization. The dense dendritic arborization is not bushlike in shape, but is flat, in the plane of the paper, like a cedar frond. Through the holelike spaces in this arborization pass millions of tiny axons, which run like telegraph wires perpendicular to the plane of the paper. The Purkinje cell's axon gives off a few initial branches close

to the cell body and then descends to cell clusters deep in the cerebellum some centimeters away, where it breaks up into numerous terminal branches. At life size, the total height of the cell (cell body plus dendrites) is about 1 millimeter. *Middle:* Ramón y Cajal made this drawing of a pyramidal cell in the cerebral cortex stained by the Golgi method. At life size, the total height of this drawing would be about 1 millimeter. Only a part of the main axon

(a) is shown: after giving off two branches (c), it might continue out of the picture for a distance of centimeters—even meters— before ending in a dense bush of branches. The cell body is the small black blob. *Right:* This drawing by Jennifer Lund shows a cortical cell that would be classed as "stellate". The dark blob in the center is the cell body. Both axons (fine) and dendrites (coarse) branch and extend up and down for a distance of 1 millimeter.

these are called *dendrites.* The entire nerve cell—the cell body, axon, and dendrites—is enclosed in the cell membrane.

The cell body and dendrites receive information from other nerve cells; the axon transmits information from the nerve cell to other nerve cells.

The axon can be anywhere from less than a millimeter to a meter or more in length; the dendrites are mostly in the millimeter range. Near the point where it ends, an axon usually splits into many branches, whose terminal parts come very close to but do not quite touch the cell bodies or dendrites of other nerve cells. At these regions, called *synapses,* information is conveyed from one nerve cell, the *presynaptic* cell, to the next, the *postsynaptic* cell.

The signals in a nerve begin at a point on the axon close to where it joins the cell body; they travel along the axon away from the cell body, finally invading the terminal branches. At a terminal, the information is transferred across the synapse to the next cell or cells by a process called *chemical transmission,* which we take up in Chapter 2.

Far from being all the same, nerve cells come in many different types. Although we see some overlap between types, on the whole the distinctiveness is what is impressive. No one knows how many types exist in the brain, but it is certainly over one hundred and could be over one thousand. No two nerve cells are identical. We can regard two cells of the same class as resembling each other about as closely as two oak or two maple trees do and regard two different classes as differing in much the same way as maples differ from oaks or even from dandelions. You should not view classes of cells as rigid divisions: whether you are a splitter or a lumper will determine whether you think of the retina and the cerebral cortex as each containing fifty types of cells or each half a dozen (see the examples on the facing page).

The connections within and between cells or groups of cells in the brain are usually not obvious, and it has taken centuries to work out the most prominent pathways. Because several bundles of fibers often streak through each other in dense meshworks, we need special methods to reveal each bundle separately. Any piece of brain we choose to examine can be packed to an incredible degree with cell bodies, dendrites, and axons, with little space between. As a result, methods of staining cells that can resolve and reveal the organization of a more loosely packed structure, such as the liver or kidney, produce only a dense black smear in the brain. But neuroanatomists have devised powerful new ways of revealing both the separate cells in a single structure and the connections between different structures.

As you might expect, neurons having similar or related functions are often interconnected. Richly interconnected cells are often grouped together in the nervous system, for the obvious reason that short axons are more efficient: they are cheaper to make, take up less room, and get their messages to their destinations faster. The brain therefore contains hundreds of aggregations of cells, which may take the form of balls or of stacks of layered plates. The cerebral cortex is an example of a single gigantic plate of cells, two millimeters thick and a square foot or so in area. Short connections can run between the neurons within a given structure, or large numbers of long fibers that form cables, or *tracts,* can run from one structure to another. The balls or plates are often connected in serial order as *pathways* (see the illustration on the next page).

A good example of such a serially connected system is the visual pathway. The retina of each eye consists of a plate having three layers of cells, one of

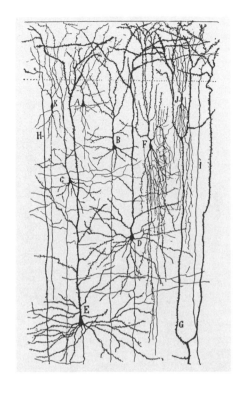

This Golgi stain, in a drawing by Ramón y Cajal, shows a few cells in the upper layers of cerebral cortex in a one-month-old human baby. Only a tiny fraction of a percent of the cells in the area have stained.

The visual pathway. Each structure, shown as a box, consists of millions of cells, aggregated into sheets. Each receives inputs from one or more structures at lower levels in the path and each sends its output to several structures at higher levels. The path has been traced only for four or five stages beyond the primary visual cortex.

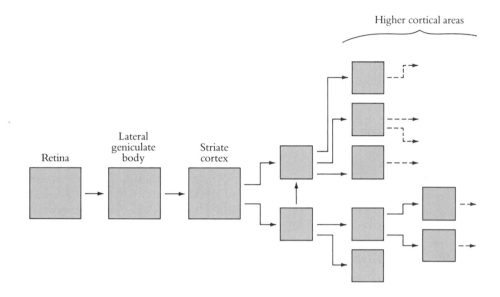

which contains the light-sensitive receptor cells, or rods and cones. As we saw earlier, each eye contains over 125 million receptors. The two retinas send their output to two peanut-size nests of cells deep within the brain, *the lateral geniculate bodies*. These structures in turn send their fibers to the visual part of the cerebral cortex. More specifically, they go to the striate cortex, or primary visual cortex. From there, after being passed from layer to layer through several sets of synaptically connected cells, the information is sent to several neighboring higher visual areas; each of these sends its output to several others (see the illustration on this page). Each of these cortical areas contains three or four synaptic stages, just as the retina did. The lobe of the brain farthest to the rear, the occipital lobe, contains at least a dozen of these visual areas (each about the size of a postage stamp), and many more seem to be housed in the parietal and temporal lobes just in front of that. Here, however, our knowledge of the path becomes vague.

Our main goal in this book will be to understand why all these chains of neuronal structures exist, how they work, and what they do. We want to know what kind of visual information travels along a trunk of fibers, and how the information is modified in each region—retina, lateral geniculate body, and the various levels of cortex. We attack the problem by using the microelectrode, the single most important tool in the modern era of neurophysiology. We insert the microelectrode (usually a fine insulated wire) into whatever structure we wish to study—for example, the lateral geniculate body—so that

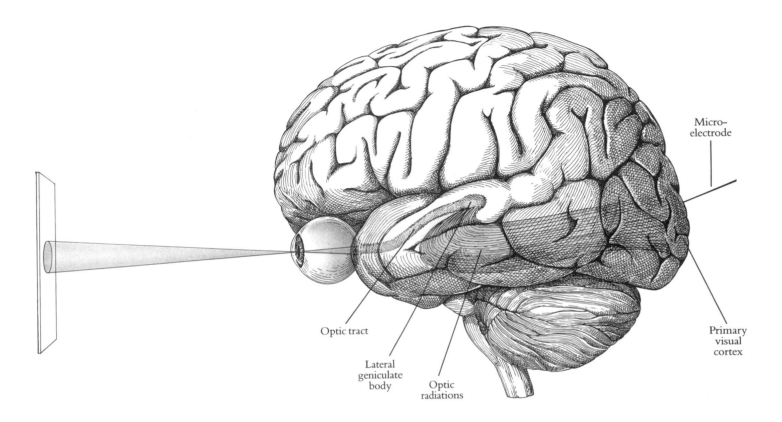

Micro-
electrode

Primary
visual
cortex

Optic tract

Lateral
geniculate
body

Optic
radiations

its tip comes close enough to a cell to pick up its electrical signals. We attempt to influence those signals by shining spots or patterns of light on the animal's retina.

Because the lateral geniculate body receives its main input from the retina, each cell in the geniculate will receive connections from rods and cones—not directly but by way of intermediate retinal cells. As you will see in Chapter 3, the population of rods and cones that feed into a given cell in the visual pathway are not scattered about all over the retina but are clustered into a small area. This area of the retina is called the *receptive field* of the cell. So our first step, in shining the light here and there on the retina, is to find the cell's receptive field. Once we have defined the receptive field's boundaries, we can begin to vary the shape, size, color, and rate of movement of the stimulus—to learn what kinds of visual stimuli cause the cell to respond best.

We do not have to shine our light directly into the retina. It is usually easier and more natural to project our stimuli onto a screen a few meters away from the animal. The eye then produces on the retina a well-focused image of the

An experimental plan for recording from the visual pathway. The animal, usually a macaque monkey, faces a screen onto which we project a stimulus. We record by inserting a microelectrode into some part of the pathway, in this case, the primary visual cortex. (The brain in this diagram is from a human, but a monkey brain is very similar.)

screen and the stimulus. We can now go ahead and determine the position, on the screen, of the receptive field's projection. If we wish, we can think of the receptive field as the part of the animal's visual world—in this case, the screen—that is seen by the cell we are recording from.

We soon learn that cells can be choosy, and usually are. It may take some time and groping before we succeed in finding a stimulus that produces a really vigorous response from the cell. At first we may have difficulty even finding the receptive field on the screen, although at early stages, such as in the geniculate, we may locate it easily. Cells in the geniculate are choosy as to the size of a spot they will respond to or as to whether it is black on a white background or white on black. At higher levels in the brain, an edge (the line produced by a light-dark boundary) may be required to evoke a response from some cells, in which case the cells are likely to be fussy about the orientation of the edge—whether it is vertical, horizontal, or oblique. It may be important whether the stimulus is stationary or moves across the retina (or screen), or whether it is colored or white. If both eyes are looking at the screen, the exact screen distance may be crucial. Different cells, even within the same structure, may differ greatly in the stimuli to which they respond. We learn everything we can think to ask about a cell, and then move the electrode forward a fraction of a millimeter to the next cell, where we start testing all over again.

From any one structure, we typically record from hundreds of cells, in experiments that take hours or days. Sooner or later we begin to form a general idea of what the cells in that structure have in common, and the ways in which they differ. Since each of these structures has millions of cells, we can sample only a small fraction of the population, but luckily there are not millions of *kinds* of cells, and sooner or later we stop finding new varieties. When we are satisfied, we take a deep breath and go on to the next level—going, for example, from the lateral geniculate body to the striate cortex—and there we repeat the whole procedure. The behavior of cells at the next stage will usually be more complicated than the behavior of cells at the previous level: the difference can be slight or it can be dramatic. By comparing successive levels, we begin to understand what each level is contributing to the analysis of our visual world—what operation each structure is performing on the information it receives so that it can extract from the environment information that is biologically useful to the animal.

By now, the striate cortex has been thoroughly studied in many laboratories. We have far less knowledge about the next cortical area, visual area 2, but there, too, we are beginning to get a fair understanding of what the cells are doing. The same is true of a third area, the middle temporal (MT) area, to which both the striate cortex and visual area 2 connect. From there on, however, our knowledge becomes rapidly more sketchy: in two or three regions we have only a vague idea of the kinds of information that are handled—things such as color or recognition of complex objects such as faces—and after that, for the dozen or so areas that we can be sure are primarily visual, we know practically nothing. But the strategy is clearly paying off, to judge from the rate at which our understanding is increasing. In the chapters to come, I will fill out some of the details of this picture for levels up to and including the striate cortex. In Chapter 2, I describe roughly how impulses and synapses work and give a few examples of neural pathways in order to illustrate some general principles of neuronal organization. From then on I will concentrate on vision, first on the anatomy and physiology of the retina, then on the physiology of the striate cortex and its anatomy. I next describe the remarkable geometric cortical patterns that result from the fact that cells with similar functions tend to aggregate together. Then will come several special topics: mechanisms for color perception and depth perception, the function of the fibers that connect the two hemispheres (the *corpus callosum*), and, finally, the influence of early experience on the visual system. Some parts of the story, such as the sections dealing with the nerve impulse and with color vision, will necessarily be slightly more technical than others. In those cases, I can only hope that you will adhere to the wise advice: "When in perplexity, read on!"

Esquema de la estructura de la retina de los mamíferos.
1. Capa de los conos y bastones. 2. Capa limitante externa. 3. Capa de los granos externos.
4. Capa plexiforme externa. 5. Capa de los granos internos. 6. Capa plexiforme interna. 7. Capa de las células ganglionares 8. Capa de las fibras del nervio óptico. 9. Capa limitante interna.

A. Células pigmentarias. B. Células epiteliales.
a. bastones. b. conos. c. núcleo de los bastones. d. núcleo de los conos. e. célula horizontal grande. f. bipolar relacionada con los conos. g. bipolar relacionada con los bastones. h. células amacrinas. i. célula ganglionar gigante. j. células ganglionares pequeñas.

This cross-sectional microscopic drawing of the nerve cells in the retina was made by Santiago Ramón y Cajal, the greatest neuroanatomist of all time. From the top, where the slender rods and fatter cones are shown, to the bottom, where optic nerve fibers lead off to the right, the retina measures one-quarter millimeter.

2

IMPULSES, SYNAPSES, AND CIRCUITS

A large part of neuroscience concerns the nuts and bolts of the subject: how single cells work and how information is conveyed from cell to cell across synapses. It should be obvious that without such knowledge we are in the position of someone who wants to understand the workings of a radio or TV but does not know anything about resistors, condensers, or transistors. In the last few decades, thanks to the ingenuity of several neurophysiologists, of whom the best known are Andrew Huxley, Alan Hodgkin, Bernard Katz, John Eccles, and Stephen Kuffler, the physicochemical mechanisms of nerve and synaptic transmission have become well understood. It should be equally obvious, however, that this kind of knowledge by itself cannot lead to an understanding of the brain, just as knowledge about resistors, condensers, and transistors alone will not make us understand a radio or TV, or knowledge of the chemistry of ink equip us to understand a Shakespeare play.

In this chapter I begin by summing up part of what we know about nerve conduction and synaptic transmission. To grasp the subject adequately, it is a great help to know some physical chemistry and electricity, but I think that anyone can get a reasonable feel for the subject without that. And in any case you only need a very rudimentary understanding of these topics to follow the subsequent chapters.

The job of a nerve cell is to take in information from the cells that feed into it, to sum up, or *integrate*, that information, and to deliver the integrated information to other cells. The information is usually conveyed in the form of brief events called *nerve impulses*. In a given cell, one impulse is the same as any other; they are stereotyped events. At any moment a cell's rate of firing impulses is determined by information it has just received from the cells feeding into it, and its firing rate conveys information to the cells that it in turn feeds into. Impulse rates vary from one every few seconds or even slower to about 1000 per second at the extreme upper limit.

THE MEMBRANE POTENTIAL

What happens when information is transferred from one cell to another at the synapse? In the first cell, an electrical signal, or *impulse*, is initiated on the part of an axon closest to the cell body. The impulse travels down the axon to its terminals. At each terminal, as a result of the impulse, a chemical is released into the narrow, fluid-filled gap between one cell and the next— the *synaptic cleft*—and diffuses across this 0.02-micrometer gap to the second, postsynaptic, cell. There it affects the membrane of the second cell in such a way as to make the second cell either more or less likely to fire impulses. That is quite a mouthful, but let's go back and examine the process in detail.

The nerve cell is bathed in and contains salt water. The salt consists not only of sodium chloride, but also of potassium chloride, calcium chloride, and a few less common salts. Because most of the salt molecules are ionized, the fluids both inside and outside the cell will contain chloride, potassium, sodium, and calcium ions (Cl^-, K^+, Na^+, and Ca^{2+}).

In the *resting state*, the inside and outside of the cell differ in electrical potential by approximately one-tenth of a volt, positive outside. The precise value is more like 0.07 volts, or 70 millivolts. The signals that the nerve conveys consist of transient changes in this resting potential, which travel along the fiber from the cell body to the axon endings. I will begin by describing how the charge across the cell membrane arises.

The nerve-cell membrane, which covers the entire neuron, is a structure of extraordinary complexity. It is not continuous, like a rubber balloon or hose, but contains millions of passages through which substances can pass from one side to the other. Some are pores, of various sizes and shapes. These are now known to be proteins in the form of tubes that span the fatty substance of the membrane from one side to the other. Some are more than just pores; they are little machine-like proteins called *pumps*, which can sieze ions of one kind and bodily eject them from the cell, while bringing others in from the outside. This pumping requires energy, which the cell ultimately gets by metabolizing glucose and oxygen. Other pores, called *channels*, are valves that can open and close. What influences a given pore to open or close depends on what kind of pore it is. Some are affected by the charge across the membrane; others open or close in response to chemicals floating around in the fluid inside or outside the cell.

The charge across the membrane at any instant is determined by the concentrations of the ions inside and out and by whether the various pores are open or closed. (I have already said that pores are affected by the charge, and now I am saying that the charge is determined by the pores. Let's just say for now that the two things can be interdependent. I will explain more soon.) Given the existence of several kinds of pores and several kinds of ions, you can see that the system is complicated. To unravel it, as Hodgkin and Huxley did in 1952, was an immense accomplishment.

First, how does the charge get there? Suppose you start with no charge across the membrane and with the concentrations of all ions equal inside and outside. Now you turn on a pump that ejects one kind of ion, say sodium, and for each ion ejected brings in another kind, say potassium. The pump will not in itself produce any charge across the membrane, because just as many positively charged ions are pumped in as are pumped out (sodium and potassium ions both having one positive charge). But now imagine that for some reason a large number of pores of one type, say the potassium pores, are opened. Potassium ions will start to flow, and the rate of flow through any given open pore will depend on the potassium concentrations: the more ions there are near a pore opening, the more will leak across, and because more potassium ions are inside than outside, more will flow out than in. With more charge leaving than entering, the outside will quickly become positive with respect to the inside. This accumulation of charge across the membrane soon tends to discourage further potassium ions from leaving the cell, because like charges repel one

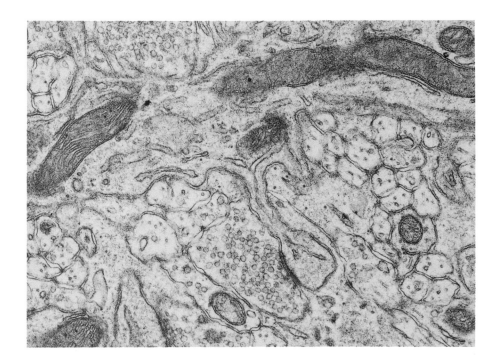

A synapse appears as the thin, dark area near the bottom center in this electron microscope picture of a section through cerebellar cortex of a rat. To the left of the synapse, an axon cut in cross section is filled with tiny round synaptic vesicles, in which neurotransmitter is stored. To the right a dendritic process (called a *spine*) can be seen coming off of a large dendritic branch, which runs horizontally across the picture near the top. (The two sausage-like dark structures in this dendrite are mitochondria.) The two membrane surfaces, of the axon and dendrite, come together at the synapse, where they are thicker and darker. A 20-nanometer cleft separates them.

another. Very quickly—before enough K^+ ions cross to produce a measurable change in the potassium concentration—the positive-outside charge builds up to the point at which it just balances the tendency of K^+ ions to leave. (There are more potassium ions just inside the pore opening, but they are repelled by the charge.) From then on, no net charge transfer occurs, and we say the system is in equilibrium. *In short, the opening of potassium pores results in a charge across the membrane, positive outside.*

Suppose, instead, we had opened the sodium pores. By repeating the argument, substituting "inside" for "outside", you can easily see that the result would be just the reverse, a negative charge outside. If we had opened both types of pores at the same time, the result would be a compromise. To calculate what the membrane potential is, we have to know the relative concentrations of the two ions and the ratios of open to closed pores for each ion—and then do some algebra.

THE IMPULSE

When the nerve is at rest, most but not all potassium channels are open, and most sodium channels are closed; the charge is consequently positive outside. During an impulse, a large number of sodium pores in a short length of the nerve fiber suddenly open, so that briefly the sodium ions dominate and that part of the nerve suddenly becomes negative outside, relative to inside. The sodium pores then reclose, and meanwhile even more potassium pores have opened than are open in the resting state. Both events—the sodium pores reclosing and additional potassium pores opening—lead to the rapid restoration of the positive-outside resting state. The whole sequence lasts about one-thousandth of a second.

All this depends on the circumstances that influence pores to open and close. For both Na^+ and K^+ channels, the pores are sensitive to the charge across the membrane. Making the membrane less positive outside—*depolarizing* it from its resting state—results in the opening of the pores. The effects are not identical for the two kinds of pores: the sodium pores, once opened, close of their own accord, even though the depolarization is maintained, and are then incapable of reopening for a few thousandths of a second; the potassium pores stay open as long as the depolarization is kept up. For a given depolarization, the number of sodium ions entering is at first greater than the number of potassium ions leaving, and the membrane swings negative outside with respect to inside; later, potassium dominates and the resting potential is restored.

In this sequence of events constituting an impulse, in which pores open, ions cross, and the membrane potential changes and changes back, the number of

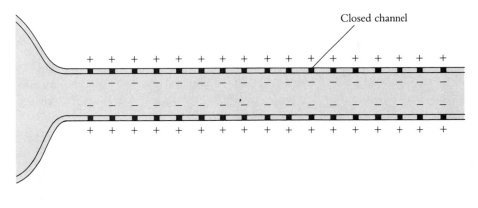

Closed channel

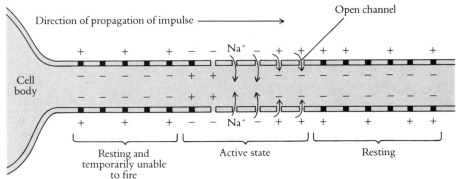

Direction of propagation of impulse ———————⟶

Open channel

Na⁺

Na⁺

Cell
body

Resting and
temporarily unable
to fire

Active state

Resting

Top: A segment of nerve axon at rest. The sodium pump has expelled most sodium ions and brought in potassium ions. Sodium channels are mainly closed. Because many potassium channels are open, enough potassium ions have left relative to those entering to charge the membrane to 70 millivolts positive outside. *Bottom:* A nerve impulse is traveling from left to right. At the extreme right the axon is still in the resting state. In the middle section the impulse is in full swing: sodium channels are open, sodium ions are pouring in (though not in nearly large enough amounts to produce any measurable changes in concentration in the course of one impulse); the membrane is now 40 millivolts, negative outside. At the extreme left the membrane is recovering. The resting potential is restored, because more potassium channels have opened (and then closed) and because sodium channels have automatically closed. Because sodium channels cannot immediately reopen, a second impulse cannot occur for about a millisecond. This explains why the impulse when under way cannot travel back toward the cell body.

ions that actually cross the membrane—sodium entering and potassium leaving—is miniscule, not nearly enough to produce a measurable change in the concentrations of ions inside or outside the cell. In several minutes a nerve might fire a thousand times, however, and that might be enough to change the concentrations, were it not that the pump is meanwhile continually ejecting sodium and bringing in potassium so as to keep the concentrations at their proper resting levels. The reason that during an impulse such small charge transfers result in such large potential swings is a simple matter of electricity: the capacitance of the membrane is low, and potential is equal to charge transferred divided by capacitance.

A depolarization of the membrane—making it less positive-outside than it is at rest—is what starts up the impulse in the first place. If, for example, we suddenly insert some sodium ions into the resting fiber, causing a small initial depolarization, a few sodium pores open as a consequence of that depolarization but because many potassium pores are already open, enough potassium can flow out to compensate and quickly restore the membrane to its resting state. But suppose that the initial charge transfer is so large, and so many sodium pores open, that more charge is brought in by sodium than can be removed by potassium: the membrane will then depolarize still further. This will cause even more sodium pores to open, and still more depolarization, and so on, in a regenerative, explosive process. When all the sodium pores have opened that *can* open, the membrane potential is reversed in sign, relative to the resting potential: instead of being 70 millivolts, positive outside, it becomes 40 millivolts, negative outside.

The reduction in potential across the membrane, with ultimate reversal of potential, doesn't take place all at once along the fiber's length, because transfer of charge requires time. It starts in one place and spreads along the fiber at a rate of 0.1 to 10 or so meters per second. At any instant there will be one active region of charge reversal, perhaps several inches long, and this reversal will be traveling away from the cell body, with still unopened channels ahead of it and reclosed channels, temporarily incapable of reopening, behind.

This event constitutes the impulse. You can see that the impulse is not at all like the current in a copper wire. No electricity or ions or anything tangible travels along the nerve, just as nothing travels from handle to point when a pair of scissors closes. (Ions do flow in and out, just as the blades of the scissors move up and down.) It is the event, the intersection of the blades of the scissors or the impulse in the nerve, that travels.

Because it takes some time before sodium channels are ready for another opening and closing, the highest rate at which a cell or axon can fire impulses is about 800 per second. Such high rates are unusual, and the rate of firing of a very active nerve fiber is usually more like 100 or 200 impulses per second.

One important feature of a nerve impulse is its *all-or-none* quality. If the original depolarization is sufficient—if it exceeds some threshold value, (going from the resting level of 70 millivolts to 40 millivolts, positive outside)—the process becomes regenerative, and reversal occurs all the way to 40 millivolts, negative outside. The magnitude of the reversed potential traveling down the nerve (that is, the impulse) is determined by the nerve itself, not by the intensity of the depolarization that originally sets it going. It is analogous to any explosive event. How fast the bullet travels has nothing to do with how hard you pull the trigger.

For many brain functions the speed of the impulse seems to be very important, and the nervous system has evolved a special mechanism for increasing it. Glial cells wrap their plasma membrane around and around the axon like a jelly roll, forming a sheath that greatly increases the effective thickness of the nerve membrane. This added thickness reduces the membrane's capacitance, and hence the amount of charge required to depolarize the nerve. The layered substance, rich in fatty material, is called *myelin*. The sheath is interrupted every few millimeters, at *nodes of Ranvier*, to allow the currents associated with the impulse to enter or leave the axon. The result is that the nerve impulse in effect jumps from one node to the next rather than traveling continuously along the membrane, which produces a great increase in conduction velocity. The fibers making up most of the large, prominent cables in the brain are myelinated, giving them a glistening white appearance on freshly cut sections. *White matter* in the brain and spinal cord consists of myelinated axons but no nerve cell bodies, dendrites, or synapses. *Grey matter* is made up mainly of cell bodies, dendrites, axon terminals, and synapses, but may contain myelinated axons.

The main gaps remaining in our understanding of the impulse, and also the main areas of present-day research on the subject, have to do with the structure and function of the protein channels.

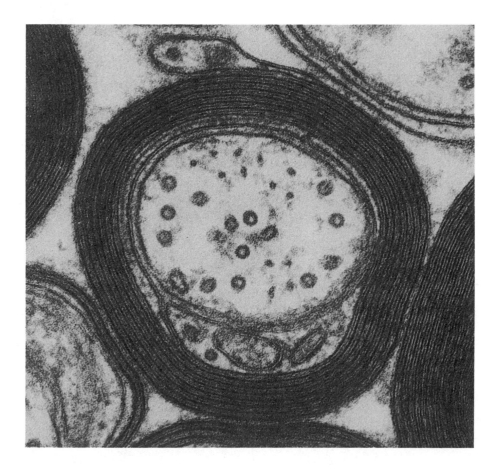

The membrane of a glial cell is wrapped around and around an axon, shown in cross section in this enlarged electron microscopic view. The encircling membrane is myelin, which speeds nerve impulses by raising the resistance and lowering the capacitance between inside and outside. The axon contains a few organelles called microtubules.

SYNAPTIC TRANSMISSION

How are impulses started up in the first place, and what happens at the far end, when an impulse reaches the end of an axon?

The part of the cell membrane at the terminal of an axon, which forms the first half of the synapse (the presynaptic membrane), is a specialized and remarkable machine. First, it contains special channels that respond to depolarization by opening and letting positively charged *calcium* ions through. Since the concentration of calcium (like that of sodium) is higher outside the cell than inside, opening the gates lets calcium flow in. In some way still not understood, this arrival of calcium inside the cell leads to the expulsion, across the membrane from inside to outside, of packages of special chemicals call *neurotransmitters*. About twenty transmitter chemicals have been identified, and to judge from the rate of new discoveries the total number may exceed fifty. Transmitter molecules are much smaller than protein molecules but are generally larger than sodium or calcium ions. Acetylcholine and noradrenaline are examples of neurotransmitters. When these molecules are released from the presynaptic terminal they quickly diffuse across the 0.02-micrometer synaptic gap to the postsynaptic membrane.

The postsynaptic membrane is likewise specialized: embedded in it are protein pores called *receptors,* which respond to the neurotransmitter by causing channels to open, allowing one or more species of ions to pass through. Just *which* ions (sodium, potassium, chloride) are allowed to pass determines whether the postsynaptic cell is itself depolarized or is stabilized and prevented from depolarizing.

To sum up so far, a nerve impulse arrives at the axon terminal and causes special neurotransmitter molecules to be released. These neurotransmitters act on the postsynaptic membrane either to lower its membrane potential or to keep its membrane potential from being lowered. If the membrane potential is lowered, the frequency of firing increases; we call such a synapse *excitatory*. If instead the membrane is stabilized at a value above threshold, impulses do not occur or occur less often; in this case, the synapse is termed *inhibitory*.

Whether a given synapse is excitatory or inhibitory depends on which neurotransmitter is released and which receptor molecules are present. Acetylcholine, the best-known transmitter, is in some synapses excitatory and in others inhibitory: it excites limb and trunk muscles but inhibits the heart. Noradrenaline is usually excitatory; gamma-amino butyric acid (GABA) is usually inhibitory. As far as we know, a given synapse remains either excitatory or inhibitory for the life of the animal.

Any one nerve cell is contacted along its dendrites and cell body by tens, hundreds, or thousands of terminals; at any instant it is thus being told by some synapses to depolarize and by others not to. An impulse coming in over an excitatory terminal will depolarize the postsynaptic cell; if an impulse comes in simultaneously over an inhibitory terminal, the effects of the two will tend to cancel each other. At any given time the level of the membrane potential is the result of all the excitatory and inhibitory influences added together. A single impulse coming into one axon terminal generally has only a miniscule effect on the next cell, and the effect lasts only a few milliseconds before it dies out. When impulses arrive at a cell from several other nerve cells, the nerve cell sums up, or integrates, their effects. If the membrane potential is sufficiently reduced—if the excitatory events occur in enough terminals and at a high enough rate—the depolarization will be enough to generate impulses, usually in the form of a repetitive train. The site of impulse initiation is usually where the axon leaves the cell body, because this happens to be where a depolarization of a given size is most likely to produce a regenerative impulse, perhaps owing to an especially high concentration of sodium channels in the membrane. The more the membrane is depolarized at this point, the greater the number of impulses initiated every second.

Almost all cells in the nervous system receive inputs from more than one other cell. This is called *convergence*. Almost all cells have axons that split many times and supply a large number of other nerve cells—perhaps hundreds or thousands. We call this *divergence*. You can easily see that without convergence and divergence the nervous system would not be worth much: an excitatory synapse that slavishly passed every impulse along to the next cell would serve no function, and an inhibitory synapse that provided the only input to a cell would have nothing to inhibit, unless the postsynaptic cell had some special mechanism to cause it to fire spontaneously.

I should make a final comment about the signals that nerve fibers transmit. Although most axons carry all-or-none impulses, some exceptions exist. If local depolarization of a nerve is subthreshold—that is, if it is insufficient to start up an explosive, all-or-none propagated impulse—it will nevertheless tend to spread along the fiber, declining with time and with distance from the place where it began. (In a propagated nerve impulse, this local spread is what brings the potential in the next, resting section of nerve membrane to the threshold level of depolarization, at which regeneration occurs.) Some axons are so short that no propagated impulse is needed; by passive spread, depolarization at the cell body or dendrites can produce enough depolarization at the synaptic terminals to cause a release of transmitter. In mammals, the cases in which information is known to be transmitted without impulses are few but important. In our retinas, two or three of the five nerve-cell types function without impulses.

An important way in which these passively conducted signals differ from impulses—besides their small and progressively diminishing amplitude—is that their size varies depending on the strength of the stimulus. They are therefore often referred to as *graded* signals. The bigger the signal, the more depolarization at the terminals, and the more transmitter released. You will remember that impulses, on the contrary, do not increase in size as the stimulus increases; instead, their repetition rate increases. And the faster an impulse fires, the more transmitter is released at the terminals. So the final result is not very different. It is popular to say that graded potentials represent an example of analog signals, and that impulse conduction, being all or none, is digital. I find this misleading, because the exact position of each impulse in a train is not in most cases of any significance. What matters is the average rate in a given time interval, not the fine details. Both kinds of signals are thus essentially analog.

A TYPICAL NEURAL PATHWAY

Now that we know something about impulses, synapses, excitation, and inhibition, we can begin to ask how nerve cells are assembled into larger structures. We can think of the central nervous system—the brain and spinal cord—as consisting of a box with an input and an output. The input exerts its effects on special nerve cells called *receptors*, cells modified to respond to what we can loosely term "outside information" rather than to synaptic inputs from other nerve cells. This information can take the form of light to our eyes; of mechanical deformation to our skin, eardrums, or semicircular canals; or of chemicals, as in our sense of smell or taste. In all these cases, the effect of the stimulus is to produce in the receptors an electrical signal and consequently a modification in the rate of neurotransmitter release at their axon terminals.

(You should not be confused by the double meaning of *receptor*; it initially meant a cell specialized to react to sensory stimuli but was later applied also to protein molecules specialized to react to neurotransmitters.)

At the other end of the nervous system we have the output: the *motor neurons*, nerves that are exceptional in that their axons end not on other nerve cells but on muscle cells. All the output of our nervous system takes the form of muscle contractions, with the minor exception of nerves that end on gland cells. This is the way, indeed the only way, we can exert an influence on our environment. Eliminate an animal's muscles and you cut it off completely from the rest of the world; equally, eliminate the input and you cut off all outside influences, again virtually converting the animal into a vegetable. An animal is, by one possible definition, an organism that reacts to outside events and that influences the outside world by its actions.

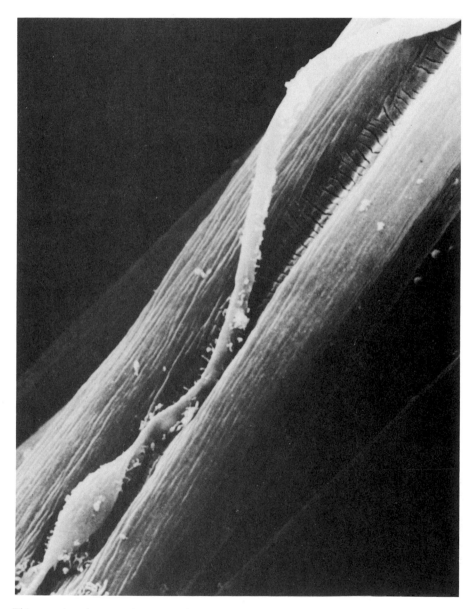

This scanning electron microscope picture
shows a neuromuscular junction in a frog.
The slender nerve fiber curls down over
two muscle fibers, with the synapse at the
lower left of the picture.

The central nervous system, lying between input cells and output cells, is the machinery that allows us to perceive, react, and remember—and it must be responsible, in the end, for our consciousness, consciences, and souls. One of the main goals in neurobiology is to learn what takes place along the way—how the information arriving at a certain group of cells is transformed and then sent on, and how the transformations make sense in terms of the successful functioning of the animal.

Although the wiring diagrams for the many subdivisions of the central nervous system vary greatly in detail, most tend to be based on the relatively simple general plan schematized in the diagram on this page. The diagram is a caricature, not to be taken literally, and subject to qualifications that I will soon discuss. On the left of the figure I show the receptors, an array of information-transducing nerves each subserving one kind of sensation such as touch, vibration, or light. We can think of these receptors as the first *stage* in some sensory pathway. Fibers from the receptors make synaptic contacts with a second array of nerve cells, the second stage in our diagram; these in turn make contact with a third stage, and so on. "Stage" is not a technical or widely applied neuroanatomical term, but we will find it useful.

Sometimes three or four of these stages are assembled together in a larger unit, which I will call a *structure,* for want of any better or widely accepted term. These structures are the aggregations of cells, usually plates or globs, that I mentioned in Chapter 1. When a structure is a plate, each of the stages forming it may be a discrete layer of cells in the plate. A good example is the retina, which has three layers of cells and, loosely speaking, three stages. When

Many parts of the central nervous system are organized in successive platelike stages. A cell in one stage receives many excitatory and inhibitory inputs from the previous stage and sends outputs to many cells at the next stage. The primary input to the nervous system is from receptors in the eyes, ears, skin, and so on, which translate outside information such as light, heat, or sound into electrical nerve signals. The output is contraction of muscles or secretions from gland cells.

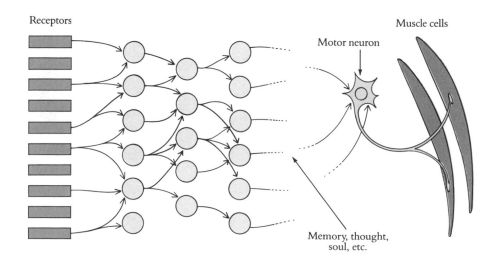

several stages are grouped to form a larger structure, the nerve fibers entering from the previous structure and those leaving to go to the next are generally grouped together into bundles, called *tracts*.

You will notice in the diagram how common divergence and convergence are: how almost as a rule the axon from a cell in a given stage splits on arriving at the next stage and ends on several or many cells, and conversely, a cell at any stage except the first receives synaptic inputs from a few or many cells in the previous stage.

We obviously need to amend and qualify this simplified diagram, but at least we have a model to qualify. We must first recognize that at the input end we have not just one but many sensory systems—vision, touch, taste, smell, and hearing—and that each system has its own sets of stages in the brain. When and where in the brain the various sets of stages are brought together, if indeed they *are* brought together, is still not clear.

In tracing one system such as the visual or auditory from the receptors further into the brain, we may find that it splits into separate subdivisions. In the case of vision, these subsystems might deal separately with eye movements, pupillary constriction, form, movement, depth, or color. Thus the whole system diverges into separate subpathways. Moreover, the subpaths may be many, and may differ widely in their lengths. On a gross scale, some paths have many structures along the way and others few. At a finer level, an axon from one stage may not go to the next stage in the series but instead may skip that stage and even the next; it may go all the way to the motor neuron. (You can think of the skipping of stages in neuroanatomy as analogous to what can happen in genealogy. The present English sovereign is not related to William the Conqueror by a unique number of generations: the number of "greats" modifying the grandfather is indeterminate because of intermarriage between nephews and aunts and even more questionable events.)

When the path from input to output is very short, we call it a *reflex*. In the visual system, the constriction of the pupil in response to light is an example of a reflex, in which the number of synapses is probably about six. In the most extreme case, the axon from a receptor ends directly on a motor neuron, so that we have, from input to output, only three cells: receptor, motor neuron, and muscle fiber, and just two synapses, in what we call a *monosynaptic reflex arc*. (Perhaps the person who coined the term did not consider the nerve-muscle junction a real synapse, or could not count to two.) That short path is activated when the doctor taps your knee with a hammer and your knee jumps. John Nicholls used to tell his classes at Harvard Medical School that there are two reasons for testing this reflex: to stall for time, and to see if you have syphilis.

At the output end, we find not only various sets of body muscles that we can voluntarily control, in the trunk, limbs, eyes, and tongue, but also sets that subserve the less voluntary or involuntary housekeeping functions, such as making our stomachs churn, our water pass or bowels move, and our sphincters (between these events) hold orifices closed.

We also need to qualify our model with respect to direction of information flow. The prevailing direction in our diagram on page 24 is obviously from left to right, from input to output, but in almost every case in which information is transferred from one stage to the next, reciprocal connections feed information back from the second stage to the first. (We can sometimes guess what such feedback might be useful for, but in almost no case do we have incisive understanding.) Finally, even within a given stage we often find a rich network of connections between neighboring cells of the same order. Thus to say that a structure contains a specific number of stages is almost always an oversimplification.

When I began working in neurology in the early 1950s, this basic plan of the nervous system was well understood. But in those days no one had any clear idea how to interpret this bucket-brigade-like handing on of information from one stage to the next. Today we know far more about the ways in which the information is transformed in some parts of the brain; in other parts we still know almost nothing. The remaining chapters of this book are devoted to the visual system, the one we understand best today. I will next try to give a preview of a few of the things we know about that system.

THE VISUAL PATHWAY

We can now adapt our earlier diagram on page 24 to fit the special case of the visual pathway. As shown in the illustration at the top of the facing page, the receptors and the next two stages are contained in the retina. The receptors are the rods and cones; the optic nerve, carrying the retina's entire output, is a bundle of axons of the third-stage retinal cells, called *retinal ganglion cells*. Between the receptors and the ganglion cells are intermediate cells, the most important of which are the *bipolar cells*. The optic nerve proceeds to a way station deep in the brain, the lateral geniculate body. After only one set of synapses, the lateral geniculate sends its output to the striate cortex, which contains three or four stages.

You can think of each of the columns in the diagram above as a plate of cells in cross section. For example, if we were to stand at the right of the page and look to the left, we would see all the cells in a layer in face-on view. Each of the columns of cells in the figure represents a two-dimensional array of cells, as shown for the rods and cones in the diagram to the side.

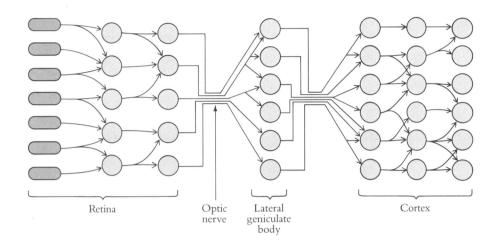

The initial stages of the mammalian visual system have the platelike organization often found in the central nervous system. The first three stages are housed in the retina; the remainder are in the brain: in the lateral geniculate bodies and the stages beyond in the cortex.

Retina — Optic nerve — Lateral geniculate body — Cortex

To speak, as I do here, of separate stages immediately raises our problem with genealogy. In the retina, as we will see in Chapter 3, the minimum number of stages between receptors and the output is certainly three, but because of two other kinds of cells, some information takes a more diverted course, with four or five stages from input to output. For the sake of convenience, the diagram ignores these detours despite their importance, and makes the wiring look simpler than it really is. When I speak of the retinal ganglion cells as "stage 3 or 4", it's not that I have forgotten how many there are.

To appreciate the kind of transfer of information that takes place in a network of this kind, we may begin by considering the behavior of a single retinal ganglion cell. We know from its anatomy that such a cell gets input from many bipolar cells—perhaps 12, 100, or 1000—and that each of these cells is in turn fed by a similar number of receptors. As a general rule, all the cells feeding into a single cell at a given stage, such as the bipolar cells that feed into a single retinal ganglion cell, are grouped closely together. In the case of the retina, the cells connected to any one cell at the next stage occupy an area 1 to 2 millimeters in diameter; they are certainly not peppered all over the retina. Another way of putting this is that none of the connections within the retina are longer than about 1 to 2 millimeters.

If we had a detailed description of all the connections in such a structure and knew enough about the cellular physiology—for example, which connections were excitatory and which inhibitory—we should in principle be able to deduce the nature of the operation on the information. In the case of the retina and the cortex, the knowledge available is nowhere near what we require. So far, the most efficient way to tackle the problem has been to record from the cells with microelectrodes and compare their inputs and outputs. In the visual

Stage 1
(rods and cones)

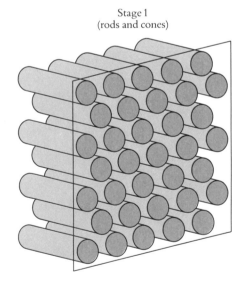

Any one stage in the diagrams on page 24 and on this page consists of a two-dimensional plate of cells. In any one stage the cells may be so densely packed that they come to lie several cells deep; they nevertheless still belong to the same stage.

system, this amounts to asking what happens in a cell such as a retinal ganglion cell or a cortical cell when the eye is exposed to a visual image.

In attempting to activate a stage-3 (retinal ganglion) cell by light, our first instinct probably would be to illuminate all the rods and cones feeding in, by shining a bright light into the eye. This is certainly what most people would have guessed in the late 1940s, when physiologists were just beginning to be aware of synaptic inhibition, and no one realized that inhibitory synapses are about as plentiful as excitatory ones. Because of inhibition, the outcome of any stimulation depends critically on exactly where the light falls and on which connections are inhibitory and which excitatory. If we want to activate the ganglion cell powerfully, stimulating all the rods and cones that are connected to it is just about the worst thing we can do. The usual consequence of stimulating with a large spot of light or, in the extreme, of bathing the retina with diffuse light, is that the cell's firing is neither speeded up nor slowed down—in short, nothing results: the cell just keeps firing at its own resting rate of about five to ten impulses per second. To increase the firing rate, we have to illuminate some particular subpopulation of the receptors, namely the ones connected to the cell (through bipolar cells) in such a way that their effects are excitatory. Illuminating only one such receptor may have hardly any detectable effect, but if we could illuminate all the receptors with excitatory effects, we could reasonably expect their summated influences to activate the cell— and in fact they do. As we will see, for most retinal ganglion cells the best stimulus turns out to be a small spot of light of just the right size, shining in just the right place. Among other things, this tells you how important a role inhibition plays in retinal function.

VOLUNTARY MOVEMENT

Although this book will concentrate on the initial, sensory stages in the nervous system, I want to mention two examples of movement, just to convey an idea of what the final stages in the diagram on page 24 may be doing.

Consider first how our eyes move. Each eye is roughly a sphere, free to move like a ball in a socket. (If the eye did not have to move it might well have evolved as a box, like an old-fashioned box camera.) Each eye has six *extraocular* muscles attached to it and moves because the appropriate ones shorten. How these muscles all attach to the eye is not important to us here, but we can easily see from the illustration that for one eye, say the right, to turn inward toward the nose, a person must relax the external rectus and contract the internal rectus muscles. If each muscle did not have some steady pull, or tone,

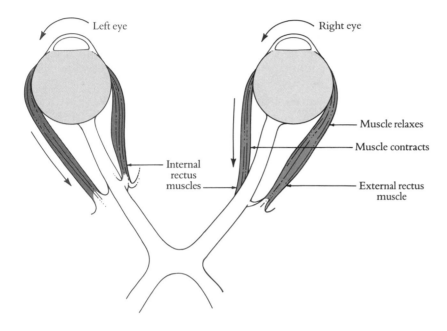

Left eye

Right eye

Muscle relaxes

Muscle contracts

Internal
rectus
muscles

External rectus
muscle

Each eye has its position controlled by six separate muscles, two of which are shown here. These, the external and internal recti, control the horizontal rotation of the eyes, in looking from left to right or from close to far. The other eight muscles, four for each eye, control elevation and depression, and rotation about an axis that in the diagram is vertical, in the plane of the paper.

the eye would be loose in its socket; consequently any eye movement is made by contracting one muscle and relaxing its opponent by just the same amount. The same is true for almost all the body's muscle movements. Furthermore, any movement of one eye is almost always part of a bigger complex of movements. If we look at an object a short distance away, the two eyes turn in; if we look to the left, the right eye turns in and the left eye turns out; if we look up or down, both eyes turn up or down together.

All this movement is directed by the brain. Each eye muscle is made to contract by the firing of motor neurons in a part of the brain called the *brainstem*. To each of the twelve muscles there corresponds a small cluster of a few hundred motor neurons in the brainstem. These clusters are called *oculomotor nuclei*. Each motor neuron in an oculomotor nucleus supplies a few muscle fibers in an eye muscle. These motor neurons in turn receive inputs from other excitatory fibers. To obtain a movement such as convergence of the eyes, we would like to have these antecedent nerves send their axon branches to the appropriate motor neurons, those supplying the two internal recti. A single such antecedent cell could have its axon split, with one branch going to one oculomotor nucleus and the other to its counterpart on the other side. At the same time we need to have another antecedent nerve cell or cells, whose axons have inhibitory endings, supply the motor neurons to the external recti to produce just the right amount of relaxation. We would like both antecedent sets of cells to fire together, to produce the contraction and relaxation simultaneously, and for that we could have one master cell or group of cells, at still another stage back in the nervous system, excite both groups. This is one way in which we can get coordinated movements involving many muscles

Practically every movement we make is the result of many muscles contracting together and many others relaxing. If you make a fist, the muscles in the front of your forearm (on the palm side of the hand) contract, as you can feel if you put your other hand on your forearm. (Most people probably think that the muscles that flex the fingers are in the hand. The hand does contain some muscles, but they happen not to be finger flexors.) As the diagram on this page shows, the forearm muscles that flex the fingers attach to the three bones of each finger by long tendons that can be seen threading their way along the front of the wrist. What may come as a surprise is that in making a fist, you also contract muscles on the *back* of your forearm. That might seem

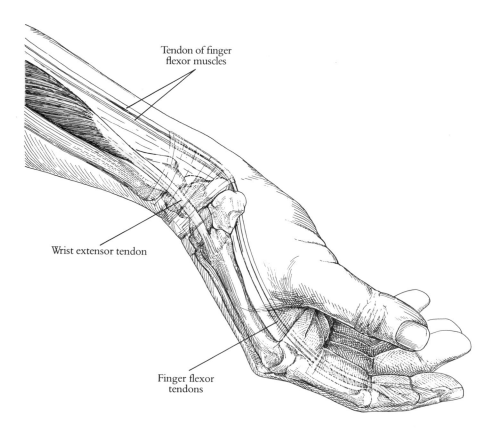

Tendon of finger
flexor muscles

Wrist extensor tendon

Finger flexor
tendons

When we flex our fingers by making a fist, the muscles responsible have to pass in front of the wrist and so tend to contract that joint too. The extensors of the wrist have to contract to offset this tendency and keep the wrist stiff.

quite unnecessary until you realize that in making a fist you want to keep your wrist stiff and in midposition: if you flexed only the finger flexor muscles, their tendons, passing in front of the wrist, would flex it too. You have to offset this tendency to unwanted wrist flexion by contracting the muscles that cock back the wrist, and these are in the back of the forearm. The point is that you do it but are unaware of it. Moreover, you don't learn to do it by attending 9 A.M. lectures or paying a coach. A newborn baby will grasp your finger and hold on tight, making a perfect fist, with no coaching or lecturing. We presumably have some executive-type cells in our spinal cords that send excitatory branches both to finger flexors and to wrist extensors and whose function is to subserve fist making. Presumably these cells are wired up completely before birth, as are the cells that allow us to turn our eyes in to look at close objects, without thinking about it or having to learn.

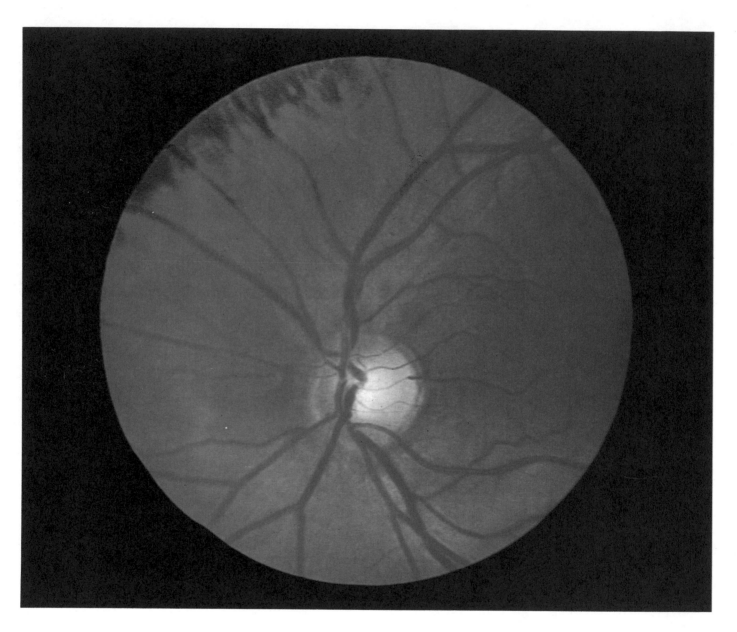

An ophthalmologist looking into the eye would see something like this photograph of a normal retina. The large pale circle is the optic disc; here arteries enter and (darker) veins leave the retina. The darker red pigmented area to the extreme right is the macula; in the center of this region, not shown, is the fovea. The black area at the upper left is normal melanin pigmentation.

3

THE EYE

The eye has often been compared to a camera. It would be more appropriate to compare it to a TV camera attached to an automatically tracking tripod—a machine that is self-focusing, adjusts automatically for light intensity, has a self-cleaning lens, and feeds into a computer with parallel-processing capabilities so advanced that engineers are only just starting to consider similar strategies for the hardware they design. The gigantic job of taking the light that falls on the two retinas and translating it into a meaningful visual scene is often curiously ignored, as though all we needed in order to see was an image of the external world perfectly focused on the retina. Although obtaining focused images is no mean task, it is modest compared with the work of the nervous system—the retina plus the brain. As we shall see in this chapter, the contribution of the retina itself is impressive. By translating light into nerve signals, it begins the job of extracting from the environment what is useful and ignoring what is redundant. No human inventions, including computer-assisted cameras, can begin to rival the eye. This chapter is mainly about the neural part of the eye—the retina—but I will begin with a short description of the eyeball, the apparatus that houses the retina and supplies it with sharp images of the outside world.

THE EYEBALL

The collective function of the nonretinal parts of the eye is to keep a focused, clear image of the outside world anchored on the two retinas. Each eye is positioned in its socket by the six small extraocular muscles mentioned in Chapter 2. That there are six for each eye is no accident; they consist of three pairs, with the muscles in each pair working in opposition, so as to take care of movements in one of three orthogonal (perpendicular) planes. For both eyes, the job of tracking an object has to be done with a precision of a few minutes of arc—or else we see double. (To see how distressing *that* can be, try looking at something and pressing on the side of one eye with your index finger.) Such precise movements require a collection of finely tuned reflexes, including those that control head position.

The cornea (the transparent front part of the eye) and lens together form the equivalent of the camera lens. About two-thirds of the bending of light necessary for focusing takes place at the air-cornea interface, where the light enters the eye. The lens of the eye supplies the remaining third of the focusing power, but its main job is to make the necessary adjustments to focus on objects at various distances. To focus a camera you change the distance between lens and film; we focus our eye not by changing the distance between lens and retina

The eyeball and the muscles that control its position. The cornea and the lens focus the light rays onto the back of the eye. The lens regulates the focusing for near and far objects by becoming more or less globular.

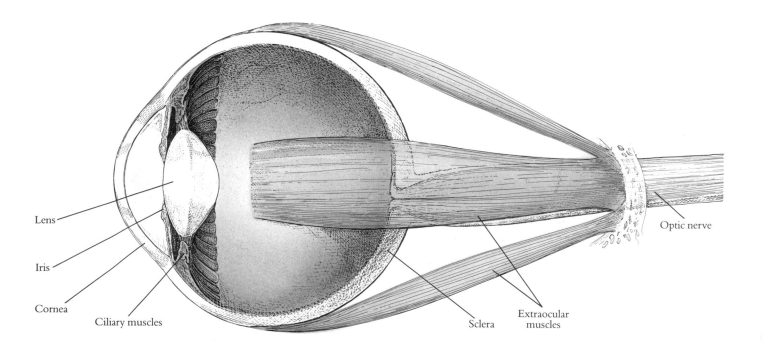

Lens

Iris

Cornea

Ciliary muscles

Sclera

Extraocular muscles

Optic nerve

but by changing the shape of the rubbery, jellylike lens—by pulling or relaxing the tendons that hold it at its margin—so that it goes from more spherical for near objects to flatter for far ones. A set of radial muscles called *ciliary muscles* produces these changes in shape. (When we get older than about 45, the lens becomes hard and we lose our power to focus. It was to circumvent this major irritation of aging that Benjamin Franklin invented bifocal spectacles.) The reflex that contracts these ciliary muscles in order to make the lens rounder depends on visual input and is closely linked to the reflex controlling the concomitant turning in of the eyes.

Two other sets of muscles change the diameter of the pupil and thus adjust the amount of light entering the eye, just as the iris diaphragm of a camera determines the f-stop. One set, with radial fibers like the spokes of a wheel, opens the pupil; the other, arranged in circles, closes it. Finally, the self-cleaning of the front of the cornea is achieved by blinking the lids and lubricating with tear glands. The cornea is richly supplied with nerves subserving touch and pain, so that the slightest irritation by dust specks sets up a reflex that leads to blinking and secreting of more tears.

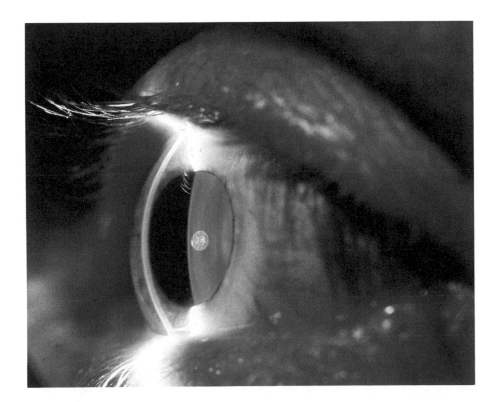

Light enters the eye through the transparent cornea, where much of the bending of light takes place. The white dot in the pupil is a reflection of light.

THE RETINA

All this intricate superstructure exists in the interests of the retina, itself an amazing structure. It translates light into nerve signals, allows us to see under conditions that range from starlight to sunlight, discriminates wavelength so that we can see colors, and provides a precision sufficient for us to detect a human hair or speck of dust a few yards away.

The retina is part of the brain, having been sequestered from it early in development but having kept its connections with the brain proper through a bundle of fibers—the optic nerve. Like many other structures in the central nervous system, the retina has the shape of a plate, in this case one about a quarter millimeter thick. It consists of three layers of nerve-cell bodies separated by two layers containing synapses made by the axons and dendrites of these cells.

The tier of cells at the back of the retina contains the light receptors, the rods and cones. Rods, which are far more numerous than cones, are responsible for our vision in dim light and are out of commission in bright light. Cones do not respond to dim light but are responsible for our ability to see fine detail and for our color vision.

The numbers of rods and cones vary markedly over the surface of the retina. In the very center, where our fine-detail vision is best, we have only cones. This rod-free area is called the *fovea* and is about half a millimeter in diameter. Cones are present throughout the retina but are most densely packed in the fovea.

Because the rods and cones are at the back of the retina, the incoming light has to go through the other two layers in order to stimulate them. We do not fully understand why the retina develops in this curious backward fashion. One possible reason is the location behind the receptors of a row of cells containing a black pigment, melanin (also found in skin). Melanin mops up the light that has passed through the retina, keeping it from being reflected back and scattering around inside the eye; it has the same function as the black paint inside a camera. The melanin-containing cells also help chemically restore the light-sensitive visual pigment in the receptors after it has been bleached by light (see Chapter 8). For both functions, the melanin pigment must be close to the receptors. If the receptors were at the front of the retina, the pigment cells would have to be between them and the next layer of nerve cells, in a region already packed with axons, dendrites, and synapses.

As it is, the layers in front of the receptors are fairly transparent and probably do not blur the image much. In the central one millimeter, however, where our vision is most acute, the consequences of even slight blurring would be disastrous, and evolution seems to have gone to some pains to alleviate it by having the other layers displaced to the side to form a ring of thicker retina,

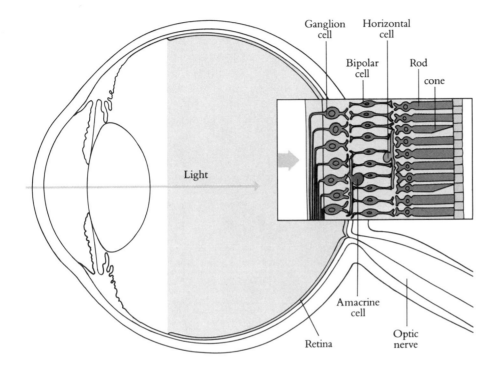

Ganglion   Horizontal
cell   cell

Bipolar   Rod
cell
                    cone

Light

Amacrine
cell

Optic
nerve

Retina

The enlarged retina at the right shows the relative positions of the three retinal layers. Surprisingly, the light has to pass through the ganglion-cell and bipolar-cell layers before it gets to the rods and cones.

exposing the central cones so that they lie at the very front. The resulting shallow pit constitutes the fovea.

Moving from back to front, we come to the middle layer of the retina, between the rods and cones and the retinal ganglion cells. This layer contains three types of nerve cells: bipolar cells, horizontal cells, and amacrine cells. *Bipolar cells* receive input from the receptors, as the diagram on this page shows, and many of them feed directly into the retinal ganglion cells. *Horizontal cells* link receptors and bipolar cells by relatively long connections that run parallel to the retinal layers; similarly, *amacrine cells* link bipolar cells and retinal ganglion cells.

The layer of cells at the front of the retina contains the *retinal ganglion cells,* whose axons pass across the surface of the retina, collect in a bundle at the optic disc, and leave the eye to form the optic nerve. Each eye contains about 125 million rods and cones but only 1 million ganglion cells. In the face of this discrepancy, we need to ask how detailed visual information can be preserved.

Examining the connections between cells in the retina can help resolve this problem. You can think of the information flow through the retina as following two paths: a direct path, from light receptors to bipolar cells to ganglion cells, and an indirect path, in which horizontal cells may be interposed between the receptors and bipolars, and amacrine cells between bipolars and retinal ganglion cells. (See the drawing of these direct and indirect connections on this page). These connections were already worked out in much detail by Ramón y Cajal around 1900. The direct path is highly specific or *compact,* in the sense that one receptor or only relatively few feed into a bipolar cell, and only one or relatively few bipolars feed into a ganglion cell. The indirect path is more diffuse, or extended, through wider lateral connections. The total area

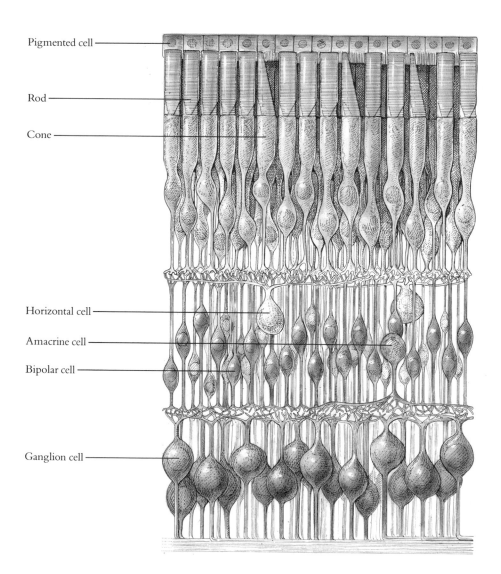

Pigmented cell

Rod

Cone

Horizontal cell

Amacrine cell

Bipolar cell

Ganglion cell

A cross section of the retina, about midway between the fovea and far periphery, where rods are more numerous than cones. From top to bottom is about one-quarter millimeter.

occupied by the receptors in the back layer that feed one ganglion cell in the front layer, directly and indirectly, is only about one millimeter. That area, as you may remember from Chapter 1, is the *receptive field* of the ganglion cell, the region of retina over which we can influence the ganglion cell's firing by light stimulation.

This general plan holds for the entire retina, but the details of connections vary markedly between the fovea, which corresponds to exactly where we are looking—our center of gaze, where our ability to make out fine detail is highest—and the far outer reaches, or periphery, where vision becomes relatively crude. Between fovea and periphery, the direct part of the path from receptor to ganglion cell changes dramatically. In and near the fovea, the rule for the direct path is that a single cone feeds a single bipolar cell, and a single bipolar in turn feeds into one ganglion cell. As we go progressively farther out, however, more receptors converge on bipolars and more bipolars converge on ganglion cells. This high degree of convergence, which we find over much of the retina, together with the very compact pathway in and near the very center, helps to explain how there can be a 125:1 ratio of receptors to optic nerve fibers without our having hopelessly crude vision.

The general scheme of the retinal path, with its direct and indirect components, was known for many years and its correlation with visual acuity long recognized before anyone understood the significance of the indirect path. An understanding suddenly became possible when the physiology of ganglion cells began to be studied.

THE RECEPTIVE FIELDS OF RETINAL GANGLION CELLS: THE OUTPUT OF THE EYE

In studying the retina we are confronted with two main problems: First, how do the rods and cones translate the light they receive into electrical, and then chemical, signals? Second, how do the subsequent cells in the next two layers—the bipolar, horizontal, amacrine, and ganglion cells—interpret this information? Before discussing the physiology of the receptors and intermediate cells, I want to jump ahead to describe the output of the retina— represented by the activity of the ganglion cells. The map of the receptive field of a cell is a powerful and convenient shorthand description of the cell's behavior, and thus of its output. Understanding it can help us to understand why the cells in the intermediate stages are wired up as they are, and will help explain the purpose of the direct and indirect paths. If we know what ganglion cells are telling the brain, we will have gone far toward understanding the entire retina.

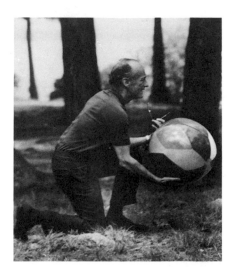

Stephen Kuffler at a laboratory picnic, taken around 1965.

Around 1950, Stephen Kuffler became the first to record the responses of retinal ganglion cells to spots of light in a mammal, the cat. He was then working at the Wilmer Institute of Ophthalmology at the Johns Hopkins Hospital. In retrospect, his choice of animals was lucky because the cat's retina seems to have neither the complexity of movement responses we find in the frog or rabbit retina nor the color complications we find in the retinas of fish, birds, or monkeys. Kuffler used an optical stimulator designed by Samuel Talbot. This optical device, a modified eye doctor's ophthalmoscope, made it possible to flood the retina with steady, weak, uniform background light and also to project small, more intense stimulus spots, while directly observing both the stimulus and the electrode tip. The background light made it possible to stimulate either rods or cones or both, because only the cones work when the prevailing illumination is very bright, and only the rods work in very dim light. Kuffler recorded extracellularly from electrodes inserted through the sclera (white of the eye) directly into the retina from the front. He had little difficulty finding retinal ganglion cells, which are just under the surface and are fairly large.

With a steady, diffuse background light, or even in utter darkness, most retinal ganglion cells kept up a steady, somewhat irregular firing of impulses, at rates of from 1 to 2 up to about 20 impulses per second. Because one might have expected the cells to be silent in complete darkness, this firing itself came as a surprise.

By searching with a small spot of light, Kuffler was able to find a region in the retina through which he could influence—increase or suppress—the retinal ganglion cell's firing. This region was the ganglion cell's receptive field. As you might expect, the receptive field was generally centered at or very near the tip of the electrode. It soon became clear that ganglion cells were of two types, and for reasons that I will soon explain, he called them *on-center cells* and *off-center cells*. An on-center cell discharged at a markedly increased rate when a small spot was turned on anywhere within a well-defined area in or near the center of the receptive field. If you listen to the discharges of such a cell over a loudspeaker, you will first hear spontaneous firing, perhaps an occasional click, and then, when the light goes on, you will hear a barrage of impulses that sounds like a machine gun firing. We call this form of response an *on response*. When Kuffler moved the spot of light a small distance away from the center of the receptive field, he discovered that the light suppressed the spontaneous firing of the cell, and that when he turned off the light the cell gave a brisk burst of impulses, lasting about 1 second. We call this entire sequence— suppression during light and discharge following light—an *off response*. Exploration of the receptive field soon showed that it was cleanly subdivided into a circular on region surrounded by a much larger ring-shaped off region.

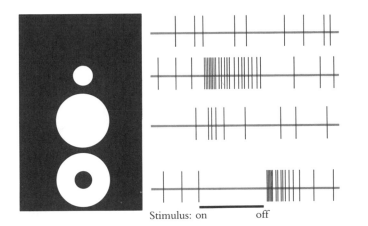
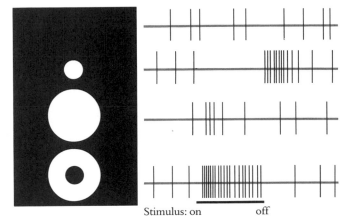

Stimulus: on   off   Stimulus: on   off

The more of a given region, on or off, the stimulus filled, the greater was the response, so that maximal on responses were obtained to just the right size circular spot, and maximal off responses to a ring of just the right dimensions (inner and outer diameters). Typical recordings of responses to such stimuli are shown on this page. The center and surround regions interacted in an antagonistic way: the effect of a spot in the center was diminished by shining a second spot in the surround—as if you were telling the cell to fire faster and slower at the same time. The most impressive demonstration of this interaction between center and surround occurred when a large spot covered the entire receptive field of the ganglion cell. This evoked a response that was much weaker than the response to a spot just filling the center; indeed, for some cells the effects of stimulating the two regions cancelled each other completely.

An *off-center* cell had just the opposite behavior. Its receptive field consisted of a small center from which off responses were obtained, and a surround that gave on responses. The two kinds of cells were intermixed and seemed to be equally common. An off-center cell discharges at its highest rate in response to a black spot on a white background, because we are now illuminating only the surround of its receptive field. In nature, dark objects are probably just as common as light ones, which may help explain why information from the retina is in the form of both on-center cells and off-center cells.

If you make a spot progressively larger, the response improves until the receptive-field center is filled, then it starts to decline as more and more of the surround is included, as you can see from the graph on the next page. With a spot covering the entire field, the center either just barely wins out over the surround, or the result is a draw. This effect explains why neurophysiologists

Left: Four recordings from a typical on-center retinal ganglion cell. Each record is a single sweep of the oscilloscope, whose duration is 2.5 seconds. For a sweep this slow, the rising and falling phases of the impulse coalesce so that each spike appears as a vertical line. To the left the stimuli are shown. In the resting state at the top, there is no stimulus: firing is slow and more or less random. The lower three records show responses to a small (optimum size) spot, a large spot covering the receptive-field center and surround, and a ring covering the surround only. *Right:* Responses of an off-center retinal ganglion cell to the same set of stimuli shown at the left.

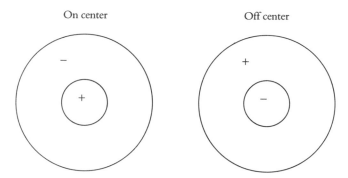

The two main types of retinal-ganglion-cell receptive fields are on center, with inhibitory surround, and off center, with excitatory surround. "+" stands for regions giving on responses, "−" for regions giving off responses.

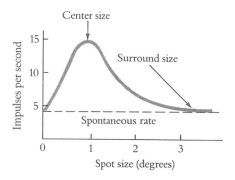

As we stimulate a single on-center retinal ganglion cell with ever larger spots, the response becomes more powerful, up to a spot size that depends on the cell—at most about 1 degree. This is the center size. Further enlargement of the spot causes a decline, because now the spot invades the antagonistic surround. Beyond about 3 degrees there is no further decline, so that 3 degrees represents the total receptive field, center plus surround.

before Kuffler had such lack of success: they had recorded from these cells but had generally used diffuse light—clearly far from the ideal stimulus.

You can imagine what a surprise it must have been to observe that shining a flashlight directly into the eye of an animal evoked such feeble responses or no response at all. Illuminating all the receptors, as a flashlight surely does, might have been expected to be the most effective stimulus, not the least. The mistake is to forget how important inhibitory synapses are in the nervous system. With nothing more than a wiring diagram such as the one on page 27, we cannot begin to predict the effects of a given stimulus on any given cell if we do not know which synapses are excitatory and which are inhibitory. In the early 1950s, when Kuffler was recording from ganglion cells, the importance of inhibition in the nervous system was just beginning to be realized.

Before I go on to describe the receptors and other retinal cells, I want to make three additional comments about receptive fields. The first is a general comment about receptive fields as a concept; the other two comments are specifically about the receptive fields of retinal ganglion cells: their overlap and their dimensions.

THE CONCEPT OF A RECEPTIVE FIELD

Narrowly defined, the term *receptive field* refers simply to the specific receptors that feed into a given cell in the nervous system, with one or more synapses intervening. In this narrower sense, and for vision, it thus refers simply to a region on the retina, but since Kuffler's time and because of his work the term has gradually come to be used in a far broader way. Retinal ganglion cells were historically the first example of cells whose receptive fields had a substructure: stimulating different parts of the receptive fields gave qualitatively different responses, and stimulating a large area resulted in cancellation of the effects of the subdivisions rather than addition. As presently used, *receptive field* tends to include a description of the substructure, or if you prefer, an account of how you have to stimulate an area to make the cell respond. When we speak of "mapping out a cell's receptive field", we often mean not simply demarcating its boundaries on the retina or the screen the animal is looking at, but also describing the substructure. As we get deeper into the central nervous system, where receptive fields tend to become more and more complex, we will find that their descriptions become increasingly elaborate.

Receptive-field maps are especially useful because they allow us to predict the behavior of a cell. In the case of retinal ganglion cells, for example, suppose we stimulate an on-center cell with a long, narrow rectangle of light, just wide enough to span the receptive-field center, and long enough to go beyond the whole field, center plus surround. We would predict from the on-center map on page 42 that such a stimulus would evoke a strong response, since it covers all the center and only a small fraction of the antagonistic surround. Furthermore, from the radial symmetry of the map we can predict that the magnitude of the cell's response will be independent of the slit's orientation. Both predictions are confirmed experimentally.

THE OVERLAP OF RECEPTIVE FIELDS

My second comment concerns the important question of what a population of cells, such as the output cells of the retina, are doing in response to light. To understand what ganglion cells, or any other cells in a sensory system are doing, we have to go at the problem in two ways. By mapping the receptive field, we ask how we need to stimulate to make one cell respond. But we also want to know how some particular retinal stimulus affects the entire population of ganglion cells. To answer the second question we need to begin by asking what two neighboring ganglion cells, sitting side by side in the retina, have in common.

The description I have given so far of ganglion-cell receptive fields could mislead you into thinking of them as forming a mosaic of nonoverlapping little circles on the retina, like the tiles on a bathroom floor. Neighboring retinal ganglion cells in fact receive their inputs from richly overlapping and usually only slightly different arrays of receptors, as shown in the diagram on this page. This is the equivalent of saying that the receptive fields almost completely overlap.

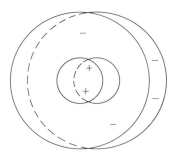

The receptive fields of two neighboring retinal ganglion cells will usually overlap. The smallest spot of light we can shine on the retina is likely to influence hundreds of ganglion cells, some off center and some on center. The spot will fall on the centers of some receptive fields and on the surrounds of others.

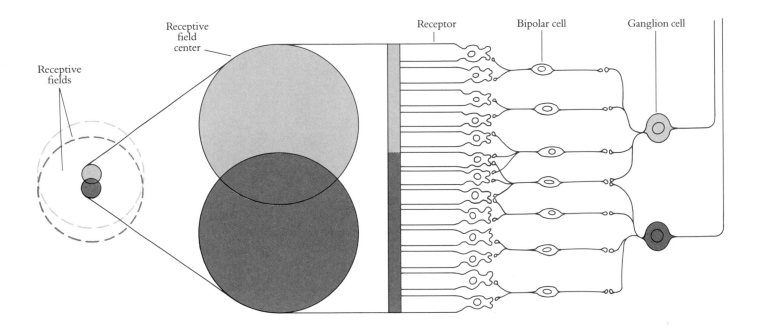

Two neighboring retinal ganglion cells receive input over the direct path from two overlapping groups of receptors. The areas of retina occupied by these receptors make up their receptive-field centers, shown face on by the large overlapping circles.

You can see why by glancing at the simplified circuit in the diagram above: the cell colored purple and the one colored blue receive inputs from the overlapping regions, shown in cross section, of the appropriate colors. Because of divergence, in which one cell makes synapses with many others at each stage, one receptor can influence hundreds or thousands of ganglion cells. It will contribute to the receptive-field centers of some cells and to the surrounds of others. It will excite some cells, through their centers if they are on-center cells and through their surrounds if they are off-center cells; and it will similarly inhibit others, through *their* centers or surrounds. Thus a small spot shining on the retina can stir up a lot of activity, in many cells.

DIMENSIONS OF RECEPTIVE FIELDS

My third comment is an attempt to relate these events in the retina to everyday vision in the outside world. Obviously our vision completely depends on information the brain receives from the eyes; all this information is conveyed to the brain by the axons of retinal ganglion cells. The finer the detail conveyed by each of these fibers, the crisper will be our image of the world.

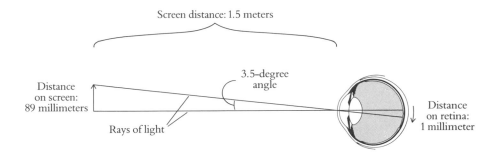

Screen distance: 1.5 meters

3.5-degree angle

Distance on screen: 89 millimeters

Rays of light

Distance on retina: 1 millimeter

One millimeter on the retina corresponds to 3.5 degrees of visual angle. On a screen 1.5 meters away, 1 millimeter on the retina thus corresponds to about 3.5 inches, or 89 millimeters.

This fineness of detail is best measured not by the overall size of receptive fields, but by the size of the field centers.

We can describe the size of a receptive field in two ways. The more straightforward description is simply its size on the retina. This has the disadvantage of being not very meaningful in the everyday scale of things. Alternatively, you could measure receptive-field size in the outside world, for example, by taking its diameter on a screen that an animal faces, but you would then have to specify how far the screen is from the animal's eyes. The way around this problem is to express receptive-field size as the *angle* subtended by the receptive field on the screen, at the animal's eye, as shown in the figure on this page. We calculate this angle in radians simply by dividing the field diameter by the screen distance, but I will use degrees: (radians × 180)/π. One millimeter on the human retina corresponds to an angle of about 3.5 degrees. At 54 inches screen distance, 1 inch on the screen corresponds to 1 degree. The moon and sun, seen from the earth, are about the same size, and each subtends one-half a degree.

Receptive fields differ in size from one ganglion cell to the next. In particular, the *centers* of the receptive fields vary markedly and systematically in size: they are smallest in the fovea, the central part of the retina, where our visual acuity—our ability to distinguish small objects—is greatest; they get progressively larger the farther out we go, and meanwhile our acuity falls off progressively.

In a monkey the smallest field centers yet measured subtend about 2 minutes of arc, or about 10 micrometers (0.01 millimeters) on the retina. These ganglion cells are in or very close to the fovea. In the fovea, cones have diameters and center-to-center spacing of about 2.5 micrometers, a figure that matches well with our visual acuity, measured in terms of our ability to separate two points as close as 0.5 minutes of arc. A circle 2.5 micrometers in diameter on the retina (subtending 0.5 minutes) corresponds to a quarter viewed from a distance of about 500 feet.

Far out in the periphery of the retina, receptive-field centers are made up of thousands of receptors and can have diameters of 1 degree or more. Thus as we go out along the retina from its center, three items correlate in an impressive way, surely not by coincidence: visual acuity falls, the size of the receptor population contributing to the direct pathway (from receptors to bipolars to ganglion cells) increases, and the sizes of receptive-field centers increase. These three trends are clues that help us understand the meaning of the direct and indirect paths from receptors to ganglion cells. The strong implication is that the center of the receptive field is determined by the direct path and the antagonistic surround by the indirect one, and that the direct path sets limits on our acuity. To obtain more evidence for this conclusion, it was necessary to record from the other cells in the retina, as I will describe in the next section.

THE PHOTORECEPTORS

It was many years before much progress was made in the physiology of the receptors, bipolars, horizontal cells, or amacrine cells. There are many reasons for this: vascular pulsations bedevil our attempts to keep microelectrodes in or close to single cells; receptors, bipolars, and horizontal cells do not fire impulses, so that recording the much smaller graded potentials requires intracellular techniques; and it is hard to be certain which of the cell types our electrode is in or near. We can circumvent some of these problems by choosing just the right animal: retinas of cold-blooded vertebrates survive when taken out of the eye and bathed in oxygenated salt water, and eliminating the blood circulation eliminates arterial pulsations; the mudpuppy (a kind of large salamander) has very large cells, easy to record from; fish, frogs, turtles, rabbits, and cats all have special advantages for one or another kind of study, so that many species have been used in the study of retinal physiology. The problem with using so many species is that the details of the organization of the retinas can differ markedly from one species to the next. Moreover, our knowledge of the primate retina, one of the most difficult to record from, has until recently had to depend largely on inferences from the results pooled from these other species. But progress in primates is accelerating as the technical difficulties are overcome.

In the past few years, our understanding of the way in which a rod or cone responds to light has dramatically increased, so much so that one has the feeling of at last beginning to understand how they work.

Rods and cones differ in a number of ways. The most important difference is in their relative sensitivity: rods are sensitive to very dim light, cones require

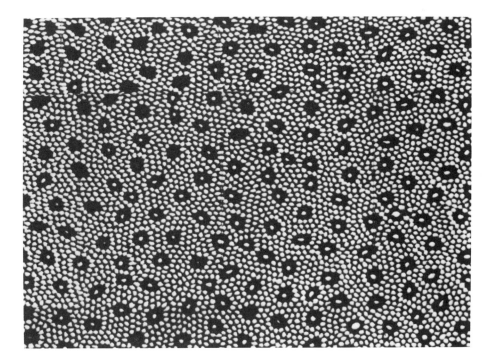

much brighter light. I have already described the differences in their distribution throughout the retina, the most notable being the absence of rods in the fovea. They differ in shape: rods are long and slender; cones are short and tapered. Both rods and cones contain light-sensitive pigments. All rods have the same pigment; cones are of three types, each type containing a different visual pigment. The four pigments are sensitive to different wavelengths of light, and in the case of the cones these differences form the basis of our color vision.

The receptors respond to light through a process called *bleaching*. In this process a molecule of visual pigment absorbs a *photon,* or single package, of visible light and is thereby chemically changed into another compound that absorbs light less well, or perhaps differs in its wavelength sensitivity. In virtually all animals, from insects to humans and even in some bacteria, this receptor pigment consists of a protein coupled to a small molecule related to vitamin A, which is the part that is chemically transformed by light. Thanks largely to the work in the 1950s of George Wald at Harvard, we now know a lot about the chemistry of bleaching and the subsequent reconstitution of visual pigments.

Most ordinary sensory receptors—chemical, thermal, or mechanical—are depolarized in response to the appropriate stimulus, just as nerves become depolarized in response to an excitatory stimulus; the depolarization leads to

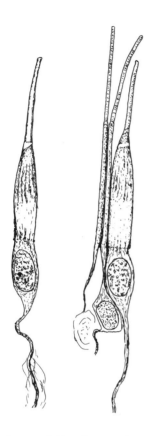

A single cone (left) and two rods and a cone (right) have been teased apart and stained with osmic acid. The slender process at the top of each cell is the outer segment, which contains the visual pigment. The fibers at the bottom go to the synaptic regions, not shown.

release of transmitter at the axon terminals. (Often, as in visual receptors, no impulse occurs, probably because the axon is very short.) Light receptors in invertebrates, from barnacles to insects, behave in this way, and up to 1964 it was assumed that a similar mechanism—depolarization in response to light—would hold for vertebrate rods and cones.

In that year Japanese neurophysiologist Tsuneo Tomita, working at Keio University in Tokyo, first succeeded in getting a microelectrode inside the cones of a fish, with a result so surprising that many contemporaries at first seriously doubted it. In the dark, the potential across the cone membrane was unexpectedly low for a nerve cell: roughly 50 millivolts rather than the usual 70 millivolts. When the cone was illuminated, this potential *increased*—the membrane became *hyper*polarized—just the reverse of what everyone had assumed would happen. In the dark, vertebrate light receptors are apparently more depolarized (and have a lower membrane potential) than ordinary resting nerve cells, and the depolarization causes a steady release of transmitter at the axon terminals, just as it would in a conventional receptor during stimulation. Light, by increasing the potential across the receptor-cell membrane (that is, by *hyperpolarizing* it), cuts down this transmitter release. Stimulation thus turns the receptors off, strange as that may seem. Tomita's discovery may help us to understand why the optic-nerve fibers of vertebrates are so active in the dark: it is the receptors that are spontaneously active; presumably, many of the bipolar and ganglion cells are simply doing what the receptors tell them to do.

In the ensuing decades, the main problems have been to learn how light leads to hyperpolarization of the receptor, especially how bleaching as little as a *single* molecule of visual pigment, by a single photon of light, can lead, in the rod, to a measureable change in membrane potential. Both processes are now reasonably well understood. Hyperpolarization by light is caused by the shutting off of a flow of ions. In darkness, part of the receptor membrane is more permeable than the rest of the membrane to sodium ions. Consequently, sodium ions continually flow into the cell there, and potassium ions flow out elsewhere. This flow of ions in the dark, or *dark current,* was discovered in 1970 by William Hagins, Richard Penn, and Shuko Yoshikami at the National Institute of Arthritis and Metabolic Diseases in Bethesda. It causes depolarization of the receptor at rest, and hence its continual activity. As a result of the bleaching of the visual pigment in response to light, the sodium pores close, the dark current decreases, and the membrane depolarization declines—the cell thus hyperpolarizes. Its rate of activity (that is, transmitter release) decreases.

Today, as a result of the work of Evgeniy Fesenko and co-workers at the Academy of Sciences in Moscow, Denis Baylor at Stanford University, King-Wai Yau of the University of Texas, and others, we are much closer to understanding the linkage between the bleaching and the closing of the sodium pores. For example, it had been very hard to imagine how the bleaching of a single molecule could lead to the closing of the millions of pores that the observed potential changes would require. It now appears that the pores of the receptor are kept open by molecules of a chemical called cyclic guanosine monophosphate, or *cGMP*. When the visual pigment molecule is bleached a cascade of events is let loose. The protein part of the bleached pigment molecule activates a large number of molecules of an enzyme called transducin; each of these in turn inactivates hundreds of cGMP molecules, with consequent closing of the pores. Thus as a result of a single pigment molecule being bleached, millions of pores close off.

All this makes it possible to explain several previously puzzling phenomena. First, we have long known that a fully dark-adapted human can see a brief flash of light so feeble that no single receptor can have received more than 1 photon of light. Calculations show that about six closely spaced rods must be stimulated, each by a photon of light, within a short time, to produce a visible flash. It now becomes clear how a single photon can excite a rod enough to make it emit a significant signal.

Second, we can now explain the inability of rods to respond to changes in illumination if the light is already bright. It seems that rods are so sensitive that at high illumination levels—for example, in sunlight—all the sodium pores are closed, and that any further increase in light can have no further effect. We say the rods are *saturated*.

Perhaps a few years from now students of biology will regard this entire story of the receptors as one more thing to learn—I hope not. To appreciate fully its impact, it helps to have spent the years wondering how the receptors could possibly work; then suddenly, in the space of a decade or less of spectacular research, it all unfolds. The sense of excitement still has not subsided.

BIPOLAR CELLS AND HORIZONTAL CELLS

Horizontal cells and bipolar cells occur, along with amacrine cells, in the middle layer of the retina. The bipolar cells occupy a strategic position in the retina, since all the signals originating in the receptors and arriving at the ganglion cells must pass through them. This means that they are a part of both the direct and indirect paths. In contrast, horizontal cells are a part of the indirect path only. As you can see from the diagram on page 152, horizontal cells are much less numerous than bipolar cells, which tend to dominate the middle layer.

Before anyone had recorded from bipolar cells, the big unknown was whether they would prove to have center-surround receptive fields, as ganglion cells do, and come in two types, on center and off center. If the answer was yes, it would almost certainly mean that the organization discovered by Kuffler for ganglion cells was a passive reflection of bipolar-cell organization. The knowledge that the receptive fields of bipolar cells were indeed center-surround and were of two types came from intracellular recordings first made by John Dowling and Frank Werblin at Harvard Biological Laboratories and by Akimichi Kaneko at Harvard Medical School. The next question is how these receptive fields are built up. To answer it we have to begin by examining the connections of receptors, bipolar cells, and horizontal cells.

The bipolar cell sends a single dendrite in the direction of the receptors. This either synapses with one receptor (always a cone) or it splits into branches that synapse with more than one receptor. When more than one receptor feeds into a single bipolar cell, they collectively occupy a relatively small area of retina. In either case, these receptors must account for the receptive-field center, because the area they occupy matches the field center in size. The next question is whether the synapses between receptors and bipolar cells are excitatory or inhibitory, or both.

To record from a cell in the nervous system is one thing: it is another to record from a cell and know exactly what kind of cell it is. This microscopic picture shows a single bipolar cell in the retina of a goldfish, recorded in 1971 by Akimichi Kaneko, then at Harvard Medical School. The fact that it is a bipolar cell and not an amacrine or horizontal cell was proven by injecting a fluorescent dye, procyon yellow, through the microelectrode. The dye spread throughout the cell, revealing its shape. In this cross section, receptors are on top.

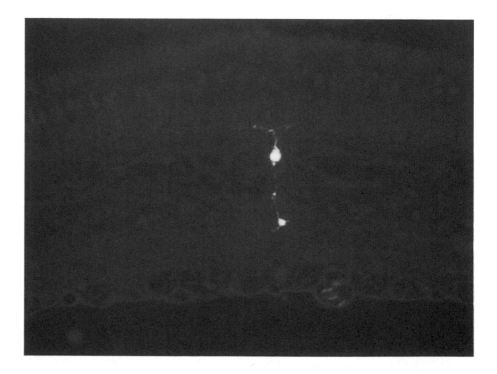

Bipolar cells, like receptors and horizontal cells, do not fire impulses, but we still speak of an on response, meaning a depolarization to light and therefore increased transmitter release from the cell's terminals, and an off response, to imply hyperpolarization and decreased release. For the off-center bipolars the synapses from the receptors must be excitatory, because the receptors themselves are turned off (hyperpolarized) by light; for the on-center bipolars the synapses must be inhibitory. To see why (if you, like me, find this confusing), you need only think about the effects of a small spot of light. Receptors are active in the dark: light hyperpolarizes them, turning them off. If the synapse is excitatory, the bipolar will have been activated in the dark, and will likewise be turned off by the stimulus. If the synapse is inhibitory, the bipolar will have been suppressed in the dark, and the light, by turning off the receptor, will relieve the suppression of the bipolar cell—that is, the bipolar cell will be activated. (No one said this would be easy.)

Whether the receptor-to-bipolar synapse is excitatory or inhibitory could depend on either the transmitter the receptor releases or the nature of the channels in the bipolar cell's postsynaptic membrane. At present no one thinks that one receptor releases two transmitters, and much evidence favors the idea that the two biolar types have different receptor molecules.

Before we discuss where the receptive-field surrounds of the bipolar cells come from, we have to consider the horizontal cells.

Horizontal cells are important because they are probably at least in part responsible for the receptive-field surrounds of retinal ganglion cells; they represent the part of the indirect pathway about which we know the most. They are large cells, and among the strangest in the nervous system. Their processes make close contact with the terminals of many photoreceptors distributed over an area that is wide compared with the area directly feeding a single bipolar cell. Every receptor contacts both types of second-order cell, bipolar and horizontal.

Horizontal cells come in several subtypes and can differ greatly from species to species; their most unusual feature, which they share with amacrine cells, is their lack of anything that looks like an ordinary axon. From the slightly simplified account of nerve cells given in the last chapter you may rightly wonder how a nerve without an axon could transmit information to other neurons. When the electron microscope began to be used in neuroanatomy, we soon realized that dendrites can, in some cases, be presynaptic, making synapses onto other neurons, usually onto their dendrites. (For that matter, axon terminals can sometimes be postsynaptic, with other axons ending on them.) The processes that come off the cell bodies of horizontal cells and amacrine cells apparently serve the functions of both axons and dendrites.

The synapses that horizontal cells make with receptors are likewise unusual, lacking the electron-microscopic features that would normally tell us which

A hypothetical circuit shows how center-surround receptive fields are thought to be built up. The receptive field center of a bipolar cell (fourth purple cell from top), an off center cell in this example, is produced by a small patch of receptors, making powerful excitatory synaptic contacts. One or several such cells feed into a ganglion cell to form its center. The surround of the bipolar cell's receptive field is produced by a much larger number of receptors (including those in the central patch), which feed a horizontal cell with excitatory synapses. The horizontal cell may contact the bipolar cell or project back onto the receptors.

If the bipolar cell is off center, the synapses onto the bipolar cell from the central patch of receptors are presumed to be excitatory. (The receptors are turned *off* by light.) The horizontal cell is presumed to inhibit either the bipolar cell or the receptors themselves. Note two input paths to ganglion cells, one directly from bipolars and the other from bipolar to amacrine to ganglion cell.

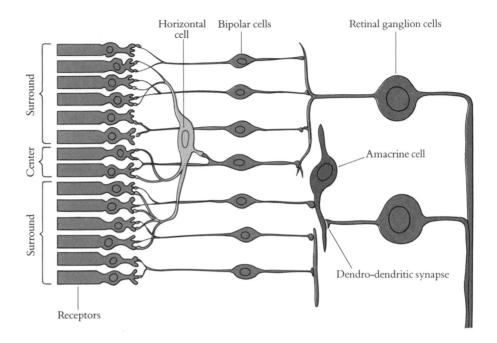

way the information is conveyed. It is clear that receptors feed information to horizontal cells through excitatory synapses because horizontal cells, like receptors, are in most cases hyperpolarized, or turned off, by light. It is less clear where the horizontal cell sends its output: in some species such as turtles we know that they feed information back to receptors; in other species they make synapses with the dendrites of bipolar cells and doubtless feed into them; in primates we do not have either type of information. In summary, horizontal cells get their input from receptors; their output is still uncertain, but is either back to receptors, or to bipolar cells, or to both.

The relatively wide retinal area over which receptors supply horizontal cells suggests that the receptive fields of horizontal cells should be large, and they are. They are about the size of the entire receptive fields of bipolar cells or ganglion cells, center plus surround. They are uniform, giving hyperpolarization wherever you stimulate, and more hyperpolarization the larger the spot. Much evidence points to the horizontal cells as being responsible for the receptive-field surrounds of the bipolar cells—indeed they are the only plausible candidates, being the only cells that connect to receptors over so wide an expanse. When horizontal cells connect directly to bipolars, the synapses to on-bipolars would have to be excitatory (for the effect of light in the surround to be inhibitory) and those to off-bipolars, inhibitory. If the influence is by way of the receptors, the synapses would have to be inhibitory.

To sum this up: Bipolar cells have center-surround receptive fields. The center is supplied by *direct* input from a small group of receptors; the surround arises from an *indirect* path stemming from a wider expanse of receptors that feed into horizontal cells, which probably feed into the bipolars. The indirect path could also be the result of the horizontal cells feeding back and inhibiting the receptors.

AMACRINE CELLS

These cells come in an astonishing variety of shapes and use an impressive number of neurotransmitters. There may be well over twenty different types. They all have in common, first, their location, with their cell bodies in the middle retinal layer and their processes in the synaptic zone between that layer and the ganglion cell layer; second, their connections, linking bipolar cells and retinal ganglion cells and thus forming an alternative, indirect route between them; and, finally, their lack of axons, compensated for by the ability of their dendrites to end presynaptically on other cells.

Amacrine cells seem to have several different functions, many of them unknown: one type of amacrine seems to play a part in specific responses to moving objects found in retinas of frogs and rabbits; another type is interposed in the path that links ganglion cells to those bipolar cells that receive rod input. Amacrines are not known to be involved in the center-surround organization of ganglion-cell receptive fields, but we cannot rule out the possibility. This leaves most of the shapes unaccounted for, and it is probably fair to say, for amacrine cells in general, that our knowledge of their anatomy far outweighs our understanding of their function.

CONNECTIONS BETWEEN BIPOLAR CELLS AND GANGLION CELLS

We have seen that the main features of the ganglion-cell receptive fields are to be found already in the bipolar cells. This leaves open the question of what transformations of information occur between bipolars and ganglion cells. It is hardly likely that nothing happens, if the complexity of the synaptic layer between the middle layer and ganglion-cell layer is any indication, for here we often find convergence between bipolars and ganglion cells in the direct path, and also the intervention of amacrine cells, whose functions are not well understood.

The synapses between bipolar cells and ganglion cells are probably all excitatory, and this means that on-center bipolar cells supply on-center ganglion cells, and off-center bipolars supply off-center ganglion cells. That simplifies the circuit: we could have had on-center cells supplying off-center cells through inhibitory synapses, for example. We should be thankful for small mercies.

Until 1976, it was not known whether on-center cells and off-center cells differed in their shapes, but in that year Ralph Nelson, Helga Kolb, and Edward Famiglietti, at the National Institutes of Health in Bethesda, recorded intracellularly from cat ganglion cells, identified them as on- or off-center, and then injected a dye through the microelectrode, staining the entire dendritic tree. When they compared the dendritic branchings in the two cell types they saw a clear difference: the two sets of dendrites terminated in two distinct sublayers within the synaptic zone between the middle and ganglion-cell layers. The off-center-cell dendrites always terminated closer to the middle layer of the retina, the on-center dendrites, farther. Other work had already shown that two classes of bipolar cells, known to have different-shaped synapses with receptors, differed also in the position of their axon terminals, one set ending where the on-center ganglion-cell dendrites terminated, the other, where the off-center dendrites terminated. It thus became possible to reconstruct the entire path from receptors to ganglion cells, for both on-center and off-center systems.

One surprising result of all this was to establish that, in the direct pathway, it is the off-center system that has excitatory synapses at each stage, from receptors to bipolars and bipolars to ganglion cells. The on-center path instead has an inhibitory receptor-to-bipolar synapse.

The separation of bipolar cells and ganglion cells into on- and off-center categories must surely have perceptual correlates. Off-center cells respond in exactly the same way to dark spots as on-center cells respond to bright spots. If we find it surprising to have separate sets of cells for handling dark and light spots, it may be because we are told by physicists, rightly, that darkness is the absence of light. But dark seems very real to us, and now we seem to find that the reality has some basis in biology. Black is as real to us as white, and just as useful. The print of the page you are reading is, after all, black.

An exactly parallel situation occurs in the realm of heat and cold. In high school physics we are amazed to learn that cold is just the absence of heat because cold seems equally real—more so if you were brought up, as I was, in frigid Montreal. The vindication of our instinct comes when we learn that we have two classes of temperature receptors in our skin, one that responds to the raising of temperature, and another to lowering. So again, biologically, cold is just as real as hot.

Many sensory systems make use of opposing pairs: hot/cold, black/white, head rotation left/head rotation right—and, as we will see in Chapter 8, yellow/blue and red/green. The reason for opposing pairs is probably related to the way in which nerves fire. In principle, one could imagine nerves with firing rates set at some high level—say, 100 impulses per second—and hence capable of firing slower or faster—down to zero or up to, say, 500—to opposite stimuli. But because impulses require metabolic energy (all the sodium that enters the nerve has to be pumped back out), probably it is more efficient for our nerve cells to be silent or to fire at low rates in the absence of a sensory stimulus, and for us to have two separate groups of cells for any given modality—one firing to less, the other to more.

THE SIGNIFICANCE OF CENTER-SURROUND FIELDS

Why should evolution go to the trouble of building up such curious entities as center-surround receptive fields? This is the same as asking what use they are to the animal. Answering such a deep question is always difficult, but we can make some reasonable guesses. The messages that the eye sends to the brain can have little to do with the absolute intensity of light shining on the retina, because the retinal ganglion cells do not respond well to changes in diffuse light. What the cell does signal is the result of a *comparison* of the amount of light hitting a certain spot on the retina with the average amount falling on the immediate surround.

We can illustrate this comparison by the following experiment. We first find an on-center cell and map out its receptive field. Then, beginning with the screen uniformly and dimly lit by a steady background light, we begin turning on and off a spot that just fills the field center, starting with the light so dim we cannot see it and gradually turning up the intensity. At a certain brightness, we begin to detect a response, and we notice that this is also the brightness at which we just begin to see the spot. If we measure both the background and the spot with a light meter, we find that the spot is about 2 percent brighter than the background. Now we repeat the procedure, but we start with the background light on the screen five times as bright. We gradually raise the intensity of the stimulating light. Again at some point we begin to detect responses, and once again, this is the brightness at which we can just see the spot of light against the new background. When we measure the stimulating light, we find that it, too, is five times as bright as previously, that is, the spot is again 2 percent brighter than the background. The conclusion is that both for us and for the cell, what counts is the relative illumination of the spot and its surround.

The cell's failure to respond well to anything but local intensity differences may seem strange, because when we look at a large, uniformly lit spot, the interior seems as vivid to us as the borders. Given its physiology, the ganglion cell reports information only from the borders of the spot; we see the interior as uniform because no ganglion cells with fields in the interior are reporting local intensity differences. The argument seems convincing enough, and yet we feel uncomfortable because, argument or no argument, the interior still looks vivid! As we encounter the same problem again and again in later chapters, we have to conclude that the nervous system often works in counter-intuitive ways. Rationally, however, we must concede that seeing the large spot by using only cells whose fields are confined to the borders—instead of tying up the entire population whose centers are distributed throughout the entire spot, borders plus interior—is the more efficient system: if you were an engineer that is probably exactly how you would design a machine. I suppose that if you did design it that way, the machine, too, would think the spot was uniformly lit.

In one way, the cell's weak responses or failure to respond to diffuse light should not come as a surprise. Anyone who has tried to take photographs without a light meter knows how bad we are at judging absolute light intensity. We are lucky if we can judge our camera setting to the nearest f-stop, a factor of *two*; to do even that we have to use our experience, noting that the day is cloudy-bright and that we are in the open shade an hour before sunset, for example, rather than just looking. But like the ganglion cell, we are very good at spatial comparisons—judging which of two neighboring regions is brighter or darker. As we have seen, we can make this comparison when the difference is only 2 percent, just as a monkey's most sensitive retinal ganglion cells can.

This system carries another major advantage in addition to efficiency. We see most objects by reflected light, from sources such as the sun or a light bulb. Despite changes in the intensity of these sources, our visual system preserves to a remarkable degree the appearance of objects. The retinal ganglion cell works to make this possible. Consider the following example: a newspaper looks roughly the same—white paper, black letters—whether we view it in a dimly lit room or out on a beach on a sunny day. Suppose, in each of these two situations, we measure the light coming to our eyes from the white paper and from one of the black letters of the headline. In the following table you can read the figures I got by going from my office out into the sun in the Harvard Medical School quadrangle:

	Outdoors	Room
White paper	120	6.0
Black letter	12	0.6

The figures by themselves are perfectly plausible. The light outside is evidently twenty times as bright as the light in the room, and the black letters reflect about one-tenth the light that white paper does. But the figures, the first time you see them, are nevertheless amazing, for they tell us that the black letter outdoors sends twice as much light to our eyes as white paper under room lights. Clearly, the appearance of black and white is not a function of the amount of light an object reflects. The important thing is the amount of light *relative* to the amount reflected by surrounding objects.

A black-and-white television set, turned off, in a normally lit room, is white or greyish white. The engineer supplies electronic mechanisms for making the screen brighter but not for making it darker, and regardless of how it looks when turned off, no part of it will ever send *less* light when it is turned on. We nevertheless know very well that it is capable of giving us nice rich blacks. The blackest part of a television picture is sending to our eyes at least the same amount of light as it sends when the set is turned off. The conclusion from all this is that "black" and "white" are more than physical concepts; they are biological terms, the result of a computation done by our retina and brain on the visual scene.

As we will see in Chapter 8, the entire argument I have made here concerning black and white applies also to color. The color of an object is determined not just by the light coming from it, but also—and to just as important a degree as in the case of black and white—by the light coming from the rest of the scene. As a result, what we see becomes independent not only of the intensity of the light source, but also of its exact wavelength composition. And again, this is done in the interests of preserving the appearance of a scene despite marked changes in the intensity or spectral composition of the light source.

CONCLUSION

The output of the eye, after two or three synapses, contains information that is far more sophisticated than the punctate representation of the world encoded in the rods and cones. What is especially interesting to me is the unexpectedness of the results, as reflected in the failure of anyone before Kuffler to guess that something like center-surround receptive fields could exist or that the optic nerve would virtually ignore anything so boring as diffuse-light levels. By the same token, no one made any guesses that even closely approximated what was to come at the next levels along the path—in the brain. It is this unpredictability that makes the brain fascinating—that plus the ingenuity of its workings once we have uncovered them.

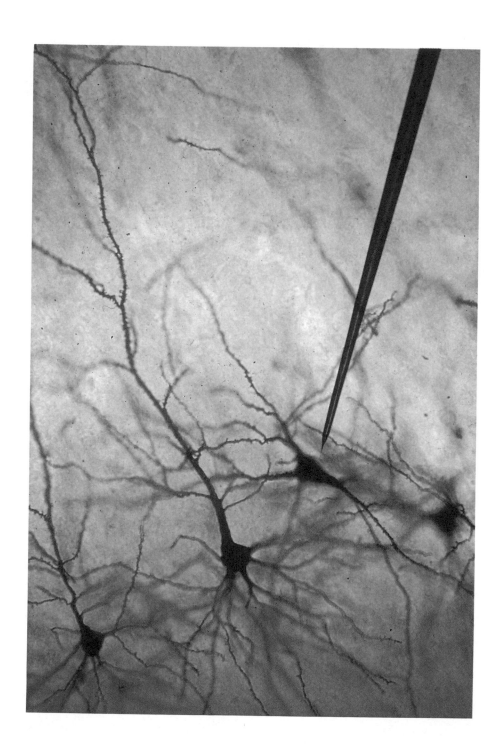

The visual cortex in a monkey, stained by
the Golgi method, shows a few pyramidal
cells—a tiny fraction of the total number in
such a section. The entire height of the
photograph represents about 1 millimeter.
A tungsten microelectrode, typical of what
is used for extracellular recordings, has
been superimposed, to the same scale.

4

THE PRIMARY VISUAL CORTEX

After Kuffler's first paper on center-surround retinal ganglion cells was published in 1952, the next steps were clear. To account for the properties of the cells, more work was needed at the retinal level. But we also needed to record from the next stages in the visual pathway, to find out how the brain interpreted the information from the eyes. Both projects faced formidable difficulties. In the case of the brain, some years were required to develop the techniques necessary to record from a single cell and observe its activity for many hours. It was even harder to learn how to influence that activity by visual stimulation.

TOPOGRAPHIC REPRESENTATION

Even before further research became possible, we were not completely ignorant about the parts of the brain involved in vision: the geography of the preliminary stages was already well mapped out (see the illustration on the next page). We knew that the optic-nerve fibers make synapses with cells in the lateral geniculate body and that the axons of lateral geniculate cells terminate in the primary visual cortex. It was also clear that these connections, from the eyes to the lateral geniculates and from the geniculates to the cortex, are *topographically organized*. By *topographic representation*, we mean that the mapping of each structure to the next is systematic: as you move along the retina from one point to another, the corresponding points in the lateral geniculate body or cortex trace a continuous path. For example, the optic nerve fibers from a given small part of the retina all go to a particular small part of

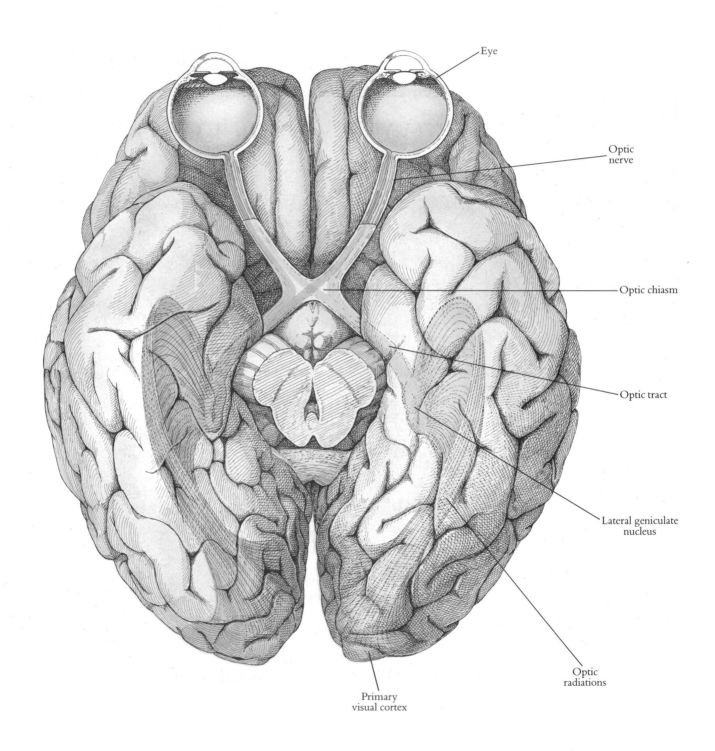

Eye

Optic
nerve

Optic chiasm

Optic tract

Lateral geniculate
nucleus

Optic
radiations

Primary
visual cortex

the lateral geniculate, and fibers from a given region of the geniculate all go to a particular region of the primary visual cortex. Such an organization is not surprising if we recall the caricature of the nervous system shown in the figure on page 24, in which cells are grouped in platelike arrays, with the plates stacked so that a cell at any particular stage gets its input from an aggregate of cells in the immediately preceding stage.

In the retina, the successive stages are in apposition, like playing cards stacked one on top of the other, so that the fibers can take a very direct route from one stage to the next. In the lateral geniculate body, the cells are obviously separated from the retina, just as, equally obviously, the cortex is in a different place from the geniculate. The style of connectivity nevertheless remains the same, with one region projecting to the next as though the successive plates were still superimposed.

The optic-nerve fibers simply gather into a bundle as they leave the eye, and when they reach the geniculate, they fan out and end in a topographically orderly way. (Oddly, between the retina and geniculate, in the optic nerve, they become almost completely scrambled, but they sort out again as they reach the geniculate.) Fibers leaving the geniculate similarly fan out into a broad band that extends back through the interior of the brain and ends in an equally orderly way in the primary visual cortex. After several synapses, when fibers leave the primary visual cortex and project to several other cortical regions, the topographic order is again preserved. Because convergence occurs at every stage, receptive fields tend to become larger: the farther along the path we go, the more fuzzy this representation-by-mapping of the outside world becomes.

An important, long-recognized piece of evidence that the pathway is topographically organized comes from clinical observation. If you damage a certain part of your primary visual cortex, you develop a local blindness, as though you had destroyed the corresponding part of your retina.

The visual world is thus systematically mapped onto the geniculate and cortex. What was not at all clear in the 1950s was what the mapping might mean. In those days it was not obvious that the brain operates on the information it receives, transforming it in such a way as to make it more useful. People had the feeling that the visual scene had made it to the brain; now the problem for the brain was to make sense of it—or perhaps it was not the brain's problem, but the mind's. The message of the next chapters will be that a structure such as the primary visual cortex does exert profound transformations on the information it receives. We still know very little about what goes on beyond this stage, and in that sense you might argue that we are not much better off. But knowing that one part of the cortex works in a rational, easily understood way gives grounds for optimism that other areas will too. Some day we may not need the word *mind* at all.

Opposite page: The visual pathway, from eyes to primary visual cortex, of a human brain, as seen from below. Information comes to the two purple-colored halves of the retinas (the right halves, because the brain is seen upside down) from the opposite half of the environment (the left visual field) and ends up in the right (purple) half of the brain. This happens because about half the optic-nerve fibers cross at the chiasm, and the rest stay uncrossed. Hence the rules: each hemisphere gets input from both eyes; a given hemisphere gets information from the opposite half of the visual world.

A microscopic cross-sectional view of the optic nerve where it leaves the eye, interrupting the retinal layers shown at the left and right. The full width of the picture is about 2 millimeters. The clear area at the top is the inside of the eye. The retinal layers, from the top down, are optic-nerve fibers (clear), the three stained layers of cells, and the black layer of melanin pigment.

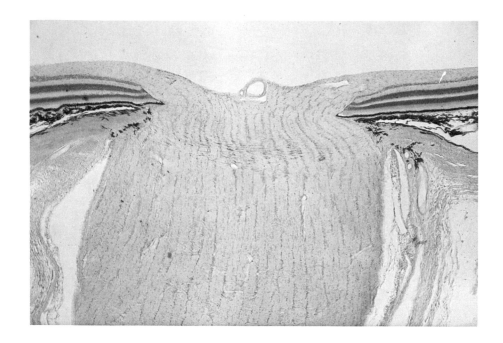

RESPONSES OF
LATERAL GENICULATE CELLS

The fibers coming to the brain from each éye pass uninterrupted through the *optic chiasm* (from *chi,* X, the Greek letter whose shape is a cross). There, about half the fibers cross to the side of the brain opposite the eye of origin, and half stay on the same side. From the chiasm the fibers continue to several destinations in the brain. Some go to structures that have to do with such specific functions as eye movements and the pupillary light reflex, but most terminate in the two lateral geniculate bodies. Compared with the cerebral cortex or with many other parts of the brain, the lateral geniculates are simple structures: all or almost all of the roughly one and one half million cells in each geniculate nucleus receive input directly from optic-nerve fibers, and most (not all) of the cells send axons on to the cerebral cortex. In this sense, the lateral geniculate bodies contain only one synaptic stage, but it would be a mistake to think of them as mere relay stations. They receive fibers not only from the optic nerves but also back from the cerebral cortex, to which they project, and from the brainstem reticular formation, which plays some role in attention or arousal. Some geniculate cells with axons less than a millimeter long do not leave the geniculate but synapse locally on other geniculate cells. Despite these complicating features, single cells in the geniculate respond to light in much the same way as retinal ganglion cells, with similar on-center and off-center receptive fields and similar responses to color. In terms of visual information, then, the lateral geniculate bodies do not seem to be exerting any profound transformation, and we simply don't yet know what to make of the nonvisual inputs and the local synaptic interconnections.

LEFT AND RIGHT
IN THE VISUAL PATHWAY

The optic fibers distribute themselves to the two lateral geniculate bodies in a special and, at first glance, strange way. Fibers from the left half of the left retina go to the geniculate on the same side, whereas fibers from the left half of the right retina cross at the optic chiasm and go to the opposite geniculate, as shown in the figure on page 60; similarly, the output of the two right half-retinas ends up in the right hemisphere. Because the retinal images are reversed by the lenses, light coming from anywhere in the right half of the visual environment projects onto the two left half-retinas, and the information is sent to the left hemisphere.

The term *visual fields* refers to the outer world, or visual environment, as seen by the two eyes. The *right visual field* means all points to the right of a vertical line through any point we are looking at, as illustrated in the diagram on this page. It is important to distinguish between *visual fields,* or what we see in the external world, and *receptive field,* which means the outer world as seen by a single cell. To reword the previous paragraph: the information from the right visual field projects onto the left hemisphere.

Much of the rest of the brain is arranged in an analogous way: for example, information about touch and pain coming from the right half of the body goes to the left hemisphere; motor control to the right side of the body comes from the left hemisphere. A massive stroke in the left side of the brain leads to paralysis and lack of sensation in the right face, arm, and leg and to loss of speech. What is less commonly known is that such a stroke generally leads also to blindness in the right half of the visual world—the right visual field—involving *both* eyes. To test for such blindness, the neurologist has the patient stand in front of him, close one eye, and look at his (the neurologist's) nose with the other eye. He then explores the patient's visual fields by waving his hand or holding a Q-tip here and there and, in the case of a left-sided stroke, can show that the patient does not see anything to the right of where he is looking. For example, as the Q-tip is held up in the air between patient and neurologist, a bit above their heads, and moved slowly from the patient's right to left, the patient sees nothing until the white cotton crosses the midline,

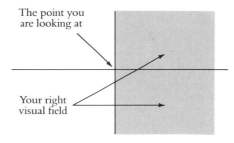

The point you are looking at

Your right visual field

The right visual field extends out to the right almost to 90 degrees, as you can easily verify by wiggling a finger and slowly moving it around to your right. It extends up 60 degrees or so, down perhaps 75 degrees and to the left, by definition, to a vertical line passing through the point you are looking at.

when it suddenly appears. The result is exactly the same when the other eye is tested. A complete right homonymous hemianopia (as neurologists call this half-blindness!) actually dissects precisely the foveal region (the center of gaze): if you look at the word *was,* riveting your gaze on the *a,* you won't see the *s,* and you will only see the left half of the *a*—an interesting if distressing experience.

We can see from such tests that each eye sends information to both hemispheres or, conversely, that each hemisphere of the brain gets input from both eyes. That may seem surprising. After my remarks about touch and pain sensation and motor control, you might have expected that the left eye would project to the right hemisphere and vice versa. But each hemisphere of the brain is dealing with the opposite half of the *environment,* not with the opposite side of the body. In fact, for the left eye to project to the right hemisphere is roughly what happens in many lower mammals such as horses and mice, and exactly what happens in lower vertebrates such as birds and amphibia. In horses and mice the eyes tend to point outward rather than straight ahead, so that most of the retina of the right eye gets its information from the right visual field, rather than from both the left and right visual fields, as is the case in forward-looking primates like ourselves. The description I have given of the visual pathway applies to mammals such as primates, whose two eyes point more or less straight ahead and therefore take in almost the same scene.

Hearing works in a loosely analogous way. Obviously, each ear is capable of taking in sound coming from either the left or the right side of a person's world. Like each eye, each ear sends auditory information to both halves of the brain roughly equally, but in hearing, as in vision, the process still tends to be lateralized: sound coming to someone's two ears from any point to the right of where he or she is facing is processed, in the brainstem, by comparing amplitudes and time of arrival at the two ears, in such a way that the responses are for the most part channeled to higher centers on the left side.

I am speaking here of early stages of information handling. By speaking or gesturing, someone standing to my right can persuade me to move my left hand, so that the information sooner or later has to get to my right hemisphere, but it must come first to my left auditory or visual cortex. Only then does it cross to the motor cortex on the other side.

Incidentally, no one knows *why* the right half of the world tends to project to the left half of the cerebral hemispheres. The rule has important exceptions: the hemispheres of our cerebellum (a part of the brain concerned largely with movement control) get input largely from the same, not the opposite, half of the world. That complicates things for the brain, since the fibers connecting the cerebellum on one side to the motor part of the cerebral cortex on the other all have to cross from one side to the other. All that can be said with assurance is that this pattern is mysterious.

LAYERING OF
THE LATERAL GENICULATE

Each lateral geniculate body is composed of six layers of cells stacked one on the other like a club sandwich. Each layer is made up of cells piled four to ten or more deep. The whole sandwich is folded along a fore-and-aft axis, giving the cross-sectional appearance shown in the illustration on this page.

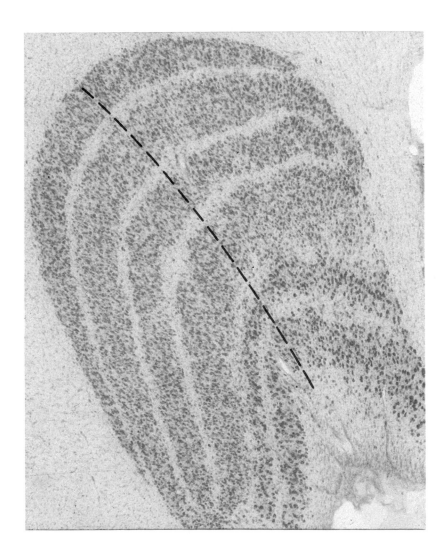

The six cell layers show clearly in the left lateral geniculate body of a macaque monkey, seen in a section cut parallel to the face. The section is stained to show cell bodies, each of which appears as a dot.

In the scheme in which one plate projects to the next, an important complication arises in the transition from retina to geniculate; here the two eyes join up, with the two separate plates of retinal ganglion cells projecting to the sextuple geniculate plate. A single cell in the lateral geniculate body does not receive convergent input from the two eyes: a cell is a right-eye cell or a left-eye cell. These two sets of cells are segregated into separate layers, so that all the cells in any one layer get input from one eye only. The layers are stacked in such a way that the eyes alternate. In the left lateral geniculate body, the sequence in going from layer to layer, from above downwards, is right, left, right, left, left, right. It is not at all clear why the sequence reverses between the fourth and fifth layers—sometimes I think it is just to make it harder to remember. We really have no good idea why there is a sequence at all.

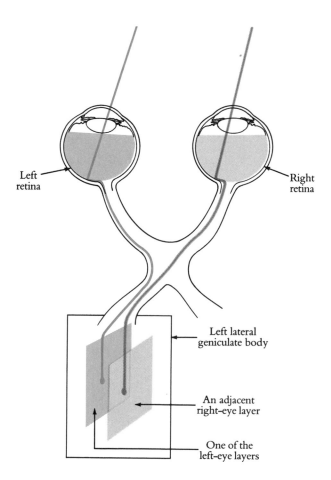

Left
retina

Right
retina

Left lateral
geniculate body

An adjacent
right-eye layer

One of the
left-eye layers

The stacked-plate organization is preserved in going from retina to geniculate, except that the fibers from the retinas are bundled into a cable and splayed out again, in an orderly way, at their geniculate destination.

As a whole, the sextuple-plate structure has just one topography. Thus the two left half-retinal surfaces project to one sextuple plate, the left lateral geniculate (see the figure on the facing page). Similarly, the right half-retinas project to the right geniculate. Any single point in one layer corresponds to a point in the animal's field of vision (via one eye or the other), and movement along the layer implies movement in the visual field along some path dictated by the visual-field-to-geniculate map. If we move instead in a direction perpendicular to the layers—for example, along the radial line in the figure on page 65—as the electrode passes from one layer to the next, the receptive fields stay in the same part of the visual field but the eyes switch—except, of course, where the sequence reverses. The half visual field maps onto each geniculate six times, three for each eye, with the maps in precise register.

The lateral geniculate body seems to be two organs in one. With some justification we can consider the ventral, or bottom, two layers (*ventral* means "belly") as an entity because the cells they contain are different from the cells in the other four layers: they are bigger and respond differently to visual stimuli. We should also consider the four dorsal, or upper, layers (*dorsal* means "back" as opposed to "belly") as a separate structure because they are histologically and physiologically so similar to each other. Because of the different sizes of their cells, these two sets of layers are called *magnocellular* (ventral) and *parvocellular* (dorsal).

Fibers from the six layers combine in a broad band called the *optic radiations,* which ascends to the primary visual cortex (see the illustration on page 60). There, the fibers fan out in a regular way and distribute themselves so as to make a single orderly map, just as the optic nerve did on reaching the geniculate. This brings us, finally, to the cortex.

RESPONSES OF CELLS
IN THE CORTEX

The main subject of this chapter is how the cells in the primary visual cortex respond to visual stimuli. The receptive fields of lateral geniculate cells have the same center-surround organization as the retinal ganglion cells that feed into them. Like retinal ganglion cells, they are distinguishable from one another chiefly by whether they have on centers or off centers, by their positions in the visual field, and by their detailed color properties. The question we now ask is whether cortical cells have the same properties as the geniculate cells that feed them, or whether they do something new. The answer, as you must already suspect, is that they indeed do something new, something so original that prior to 1958, when cortical cells were first studied with patterned light stimulation, no one had remotely predicted it.

The primary visual, or striate, cortex is a plate of cells 2 millimeters thick, with a surface area of a few square inches. Numbers may help to convey an impression of the vastness of this structure: compared with the geniculate, which has 1.5 million cells, the striate cortex contains something like 200 million cells. Its structure is intricate and fascinating, but we don't need to know the details to appreciate how this part of the brain transforms the incoming visual information. We will look at the anatomy more closely when I discuss functional architecture in the next chapter.

I have already mentioned that the flow of information in the cortex takes place over several loosely defined stages. At the first stage, most cells respond like geniculate cells. Their receptive fields have circular symmetry, which means that a line or edge produces the same response regardless of how it is oriented. The tiny, closely packed cells at this stage are not easy to record from, and it is still unclear whether their responses differ at all from the responses of geniculate cells, just as it is unclear whether the responses of retinal ganglion cells and geniculate cells differ. The complexity of the histology (the microscopic anatomy) of both geniculate and cortex certainly leads you to expect differences if you compare the right things, but it can be hard to know just what the "right things" are.

This point is even more important when it comes to the responses of the cells at the next stage in the cortex, which presumably get their input from the center-surround cortical cells in the first stage. At first, it was not at all easy to

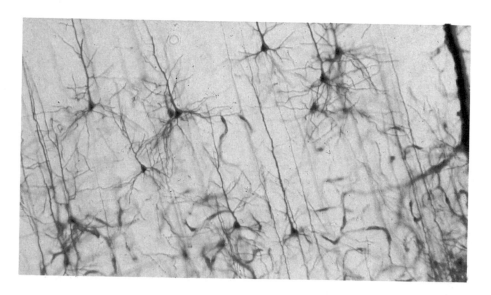

This Golgi-stained section of the primary visual cortex shows over a dozen pyramidal cells—still just a tiny fraction of the total number in such a section. The height of the section is about 1 millimeter. (The long trunk near the right edge is a blood vessel.)

know what these second-stage cells responded to. By the late 1950s very few scientists had attempted to record from single cells in the visual cortex, and those who did had come up with disappointing results. They found that cells in the visual cortex seemed to work very much like cells in the retina: they found on cells and off cells, plus an additional class that did not seem to respond to light at all. In the face of the obviously fiendish complexity of the cortex's anatomy, it was puzzling to find the physiology so boring.

The explanation, in retrospect, is very clear. First, the stimulus was inadequate: to activate cells in the cortex, the usual custom was simply to flood the retina with diffuse light, a stimulus that is far from optimal even in the retina, as Kuffler had shown ten years previously. For most cortical cells, flooding the retina in this way is not only not optimal—it is completely without effect. Whereas many geniculate cells respond to diffuse white light, even if weakly, cortical cells, even those first-stage cells that resemble geniculate cells, give virtually no responses. One's first intuition, that the best way to activate a visual cell is to activate all the receptors in the retina, was evidently seriously off the mark. Second, and still more ironic, it turned out that the cortical cells that did give on or off responses were in fact not cells at all but merely axons coming in from the lateral geniculate body. The cortical cells were not responding at all! They were much too choosy to pay attention to anything as crude as diffuse light.

This was the situation in 1958, when Torsten Wiesel and I made one of our first technically successful recordings from the cortex of a cat. The position of microelectrode tip, relative to the cortex, was unusually stable, so much so that we were able to listen in on one cell for a period of about nine hours. We tried everything short of standing on our heads to get it to fire. (It did fire spontaneously from time to time, as most cortical cells do, but we had a hard time convincing ourselves that our stimuli had caused any of that activity.) After some hours we began to have a vague feeling that shining light in one particular part of the retina was evoking some response, so we tried concentrating our efforts there. To stimulate, we were using mostly white circular spots and black spots. For black spots, we would take a 1-by-2-inch glass microscope slide, onto which we had glued an opaque black dot, and shove it into a slot in the optical instrument Samuel Talbot had designed to project images on the retina. For white spots, we used a slide of the same size made of brass with a small hole drilled through it. (Research was cheaper in those days.) After about five hours of struggle, we suddenly had the impression that the glass with the dot was occasionally producing a response, but the response seemed to have little to do with the dot. Eventually we caught on: it was the sharp but faint shadow cast by the edge of the glass as we slid it into the slot that was doing the trick. We soon convinced ourselves that the edge worked only when its shadow was swept across one small part of the retina and that

Responses of one of the first orientation-specific cells Torsten Wiesel and I recorded, from a cat striate cortex in 1958. This cell not only responds exclusively to a moving slit in an eleven o'clock orientation but also responds to movement right and up, but hardly at all to movement left and down.

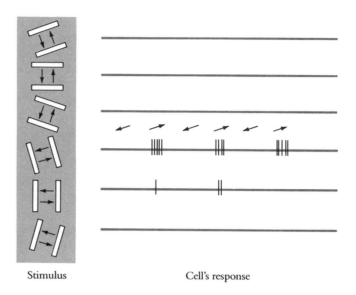

Stimulus   Cell's response

the sweeping had to be done with the edge in one particular orientation. Most amazing was the contrast between the machine-gun discharge when the orientation of the stimulus was just right and the utter lack of a response if we changed the orientation or simply shined a bright flashlight into the cat's eyes.

The discovery was just the beginning, and for some time we were very confused because, as luck would have it, the cell was of a type that we came later to call *complex,* and it lay two stages beyond the initial, center-surround cortical stage. Although complex cells are the commonest type in the striate cortex, they are hard to comprehend if you haven't seen the intervening type.

Beyond the first, center-surround stage, cells in the monkey cortex indeed respond in a radically different way. Small spots generally produce weak responses or none. To evoke a response, we first have to find the appropriate part of the visual field to stimulate, that is, the appropriate part of the screen that the animal is facing: we have to find the receptive field of the cell. It then turns out that the most effective way to influence a cell is to sweep some kind of line across the receptive field, in a direction perpendicular to the line's orientation. The line can be light on a dark background (a slit) or a dark bar on a white background or an edge boundary between dark and light. Some cells prefer one of these stimuli over the other two, often very strongly; others respond about equally well to all three types of stimuli. What is critical is the orientation of the line: a typical cell responds best to some optimum stimulus orientation; the response, measured in the number of impulses as the receptive field is crossed, falls off over about 10 to 20 degrees to either side of the optimum, and outside that range it declines steeply to zero (see the illustration on the facing page). A range of 10 to 20 degrees may seem imprecise, until you remember that the difference between one o'clock and two o'clock is 30 degrees. A typical orientation-selective cell does not respond at all when the line is oriented 90 degrees to the optimal.

Unlike cells at earlier stages in the visual path, these orientation-specific cells respond far better to a moving than to a stationary line. That is why, in the diagram on the facing page, we stimulate by sweeping the line over the receptive field. Flashing a stationary line on and off often evokes weak responses, and when it does, we find that the preferred orientation is always the same as when the line is moved.

In many cells, perhaps one-fifth of the population, moving the stimulus brings out another kind of specific response. Instead of firing equally well to both movements, back and forth, many cells will consistently respond better to one of the two directions. One movement may even produce a strong response and the reverse movement none or almost none, as illustrated in the figure on the facing page.

In a single experiment we can test the responses of 200 to 300 cells simply by learning all about one cell and then pushing the electrode ahead to the next cell to study it. Because once you have inserted the delicate electrode you obviously can't move it sideways without destroying it or the even more delicate cortex, this technique limits your examination to cells lying in a straight line. Fifty cells per millimeter of penetration is about the maximum we can get with present methods. When the orientation preferences of a few hundred or a thousand cells are examined, all orientations turn out to be about equally represented—vertical, horizontal, and every possible oblique. Considering the nature of the world we look at, containing as it does trees and horizons, the question arises whether any particular orientations, such as vertical and horizontal, are better represented than the others. Answers differ with different laboratory results, but everyone agrees that if biases do exist, they must be small—small enough to require statistics to discern them, which may mean they are negligible!

In the monkey striate cortex, about 70 to 80 percent of cells have this property of orientation specificity. In the cat, all cortical cells seem to be orientation selective, even those with direct geniculate input.

We find striking differences among orientation-specific cells, not just in optimum stimulus orientation or in the position of the receptive field on the retina, but in the way cells behave. The most useful distinction is between two classes of cells: *simple* and *complex*. As their names suggest, the two types differ in the complexity of their behavior, and we make the reasonable assumption that the cells with the simpler behavior are closer in the circuit to the input of the cortex.

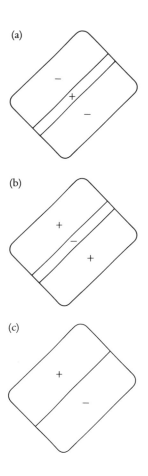

(a)

(b)

(c)

Three typical receptive-field maps for simple cells. The effective stimuli for these cells are (a) a slit covering the plus (+) region, (b) a dark line covering the minus (−) region, and (c) a light-dark edge falling on the boundary between plus and minus.

SIMPLE CELLS

For the most part, we can predict the responses of simple cells to complicated shapes from their responses to small-spot stimuli. Like retinal ganglion cells, geniculate cells, and circularly symmetric cortical cells, each simple cell has a small, clearly delineated receptive field within which a small spot of light produces either on or off responses, depending on where in the field the spot falls. The difference between these cells and cells at earlier levels is in the geometry of the maps of excitation and inhibition. Cells at earlier stages have maps with circular symmetry, consisting of one region, on or off, surrounded by the opponent region, off or on. Cortical simple cells are more complicated. The excitatory and inhibitory domains are always separated by a straight line or by two parallel lines, as shown in the three drawings on this page. Of the various possibilities, the most common is the one in which a long, narrow region giving excitation is flanked on both sides by larger regions giving inhibition, as shown in the first drawing (a).

To test the predictive value of the maps made with small spots, we can now try other shapes. We soon learn that the more of a region a stimulus fills, the stronger is the resultant excitation or inhibition; that is, we find *spatial summation* of effects. We also find *antagonism,* in which we get a mutual cancellation of responses on stimulating two opposing regions at the same time. Thus for a cell with a receptive-field map like that shown in the first drawing (a), a long, narrow slit is the most potent stimulus, provided it is positioned and oriented so as to cover the excitatory part of the field without invading the inhibitory part (see the illustration on the facing page). Even the slightest misorientation causes the slit to miss some of the excitatory area and to invade the antagonistic inhibitory part, with a consequent decline in response.

In the second and third figures (b and c) of the diagram on this page, we see two other kinds of simple cells: these respond best to dark lines and to dark/light edges, with the same sensitivity to the orientation of the stimulus. For all three types, diffuse light evokes no response at all. The mutual cancellation is obviously very precise, reminiscent of the acid-base titrations we all did in high school chemistry labs. Already, then, we can see a marked diversity in cortical cells. Among simple cells, we find three or four different geometries, for each of which we find every possible orientation and all possible visual-field positions.

The size of a simple-cell receptive field depends on its position in the retina relative to the fovea, but even in a given part of the retina, we find some variation in size. The smallest fields, in and near the fovea, are about one-quarter degree by one-quarter degree in total size; for a cell of the type shown in diagrams a or b in the figure on this page, the center region has a width of

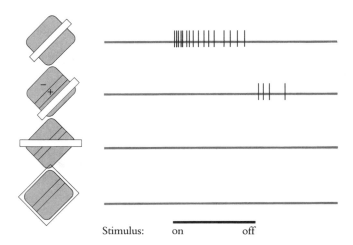

Stimulus: on   off

Various stimulus geometries evoke different responses in a cell with receptive field of the type in diagram a of the previous figure. The stimulus line at the bottom indicates when the slit is turned on and, 1 second later, turned off. The top record shows the response to a slit of optimum size, position, and orientation. In the second record, the same slit covers only part of an inhibitory area. (Because this cell has no spontaneous activity to suppress, only an off discharge is seen.) In the third record, the slit is oriented so as to cover only a small part of the excitatory region and a proportionally small part of the inhibitory region; the cell fails to respond. In the bottom record, the whole receptive field is illuminated; again, there is no response.

as little as a few minutes of arc. This is the same as the diameters of the smallest receptive-field centers in retinal ganglion cells or geniculate cells. In the far retinal periphery, simple-cell receptive fields can be about 1 degree by 1 degree.

Even after twenty years we still do not know how the inputs to cortical cells are wired in order to bring about this behavior. Several plausible circuits have been proposed, and it may well be that one of them, or several in combination, will turn out to be correct. Simple cells must be built up from the antecedent cells with circular fields; by far the simplest proposal is that a simple cell receives direct excitatory input from many cells at the previous stage, cells whose receptive-field centers are distributed along a line in the visual field, as shown in the diagram on the next page.

It seems slightly more difficult to wire up a cell that is selectively responsive to edges, as shown in the third drawing (c) on the facing page. One workable scheme would be to have the cell receive inputs from two sets of antecedent cells having their field centers arranged on opposite sides of a line, on-center cells on one side, off-center cells on the other, all making excitatory connections. In all these proposed circuits, excitatory input from an off-center cell is logically equivalent to inhibitory input from an on-center cell, provided we assume that the off-center cell is spontaneously active.

Working out the exact mechanism for building up simple cells will not be easy. For any one cell we need to know what kinds of cells feed in information—for example, the details of their receptive fields, including position, orientation if any, and whether on or off center—and whether they supply excita-

This type of wiring could produce a simple-cell receptive field. On the right, four cells are shown making excitatory synaptic connections with a cell of higher order. Each of the lower-order cells has a radially symmetric receptive field with on-center and off-surround, illustrated by the left side of the diagram. The centers of these fields lie along a line. If we suppose that many more than four center-surround cells are connected with the simple cell, all with their field centers overlapped along this line, the receptive field of the simple cell will consist of a long, narrow excitatory region with inhibitory flanks. Avoiding receptive-field terminology, we can say that stimulating with a small spot anywhere in this long, narrow rectangle will strongly activate one or a few of the center-surround cells and in turn excite the simple cell, although only weakly. Stimulating with a long, narrow slit will activate all the center-surround cells, producing a strong response in the simple cell.

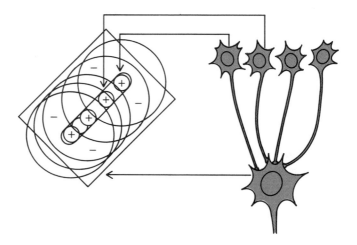

tion or inhibition to the cell. Because methods for obtaining this kind of knowledge don't yet exist, we are forced to use less direct approaches, with correspondingly higher chances of being wrong. The mechanism summarized in the diagram on this page seems to me the most likely because it is the most simple.

COMPLEX CELLS

Complex cells represent the next step or steps in the analysis. They are the commonest cells in the striate cortex—a guess would be that they make up three-quarters of the population. The first oriented cell Wiesel and I recorded—the one that responded to the edge of the glass slide—was in retrospect almost certainly a complex cell.

Complex cells share with simple cells the quality of responding only to specifically oriented lines. Like simple cells, they respond over a limited region of the visual field; unlike simple cells, their behavior cannot be explained by a neat subdivision of the receptive field into excitatory and inhibitory regions. Turning a small stationary spot on or off seldom produces a response, and even an appropriately oriented stationary slit or edge tends to give no response or only weak, unsustained responses of the same type everywhere—at the onset or turning off of the stimulus or both. But if the properly oriented line is swept across the receptive field, the result is a well-sustained barrage of impulses, from the instant the line enters the field until it leaves (see the cell-response diagram on page 70). By contrast, to evoke sustained responses from a simple cell, a stationary line must be critically oriented *and* critically positioned; a moving line evokes only a brief response at the moment it crosses a boundary from an inhibitory to an excitatory region or during the brief time it covers the excitatory region. Complex cells that do react to stationary slits, bars, or edges fire regardless of where the line is placed in the receptive field, as long as the orientation is appropriate. But over the same region, an inappropriately oriented line is ineffective, as shown in the illustration on this page.

The diagram on this page for the complex cell and the one on page 73 for the simple cell illustrate the essential difference between the two types: for a simple cell, the extremely narrow range of positions over which an optimally oriented line evokes a response; for a complex cell, the responses to a properly oriented line wherever it is placed in the receptive field. This behavior is related to the explicit on and off regions of a simple cell and to the lack of such regions in a complex cell. The complex cell generalizes the responsiveness to a line over a wider territory.

Complex cells tend to have larger receptive fields than simple cells, but not very much larger. A typical complex receptive field in the fovea of the macaque monkey would be about one-half degree by one-half degree. The optimum stimulus width is about the same for simple cells and complex cells—in the fovea, about 2 minutes of arc. The complex cell's resolving power, or acuity, is thus the same as the simple cell's.

As in the case of the simple cell, we do not know exactly how complex cells are built up. But, again, it is easy to propose plausible schemes, and the sim-

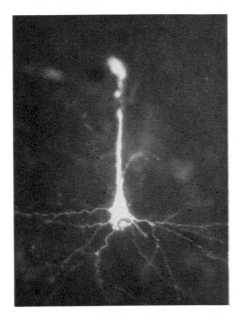

This cortical cell from layer 5 in the striate cortex of a cat was recorded intracellularly by David Van Essen and James Kelly at Harvard Medical School in 1973, and its complex receptive field was mapped. They then injected procyon yellow dye and showed that the cell was pyramidal.

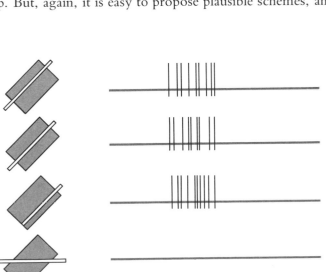

Stimulus: on   off

A long, narrow slit of light evokes a response wherever it is placed within the receptive field (rectangle) of a complex cell, provided the orientation is correct (upper three records). A nonoptimal orientation gives a weaker response or none at all (lower record).

This wiring diagram would account for the properties of a complex cell. As in the figure on page 74, we suppose that a large number of simple cells (only three are shown here) make excitatory synapses with a single complex cell. Each simple cell responds optimally to a vertically oriented edge with light to the right, and the receptive fields are scattered in overlapping fashion throughout the rectangle. An edge falling anywhere within the rectangle evokes a response from a few simple cells, and this in turn evokes a response in the complex cell. Because there is adaptation at the synapses, only a moving stimulus will keep up a steady bombardment of the complex cell.

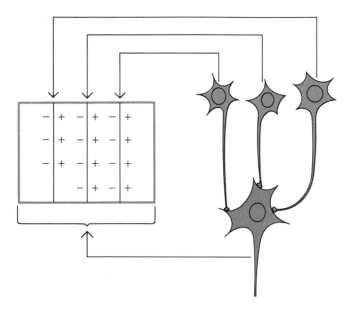

plest one is to imagine that the complex cell receives input from many simple cells, all of whose fields have the same orientation but are spread out in overlapping fashion over the entire field of the complex cell, as shown in the illustration on this page. If the connections from simple to complex cells are excitatory, then wherever a line falls in the field, *some* simple cells are activated; the complex cell will therefore be activated. If, on the other hand, a stimulus fills the entire receptive field, none of the simple cells will be activated, and the complex cell won't be activated.

The burst of impulses from a complex cell to turning on a stationary line and not moving it is generally brief even if the light is kept on: we say that the response *adapts*. When we move the line through the complex cell's receptive field, the sustained response may be the result of overcoming the adaptation, by bringing in new simple cells one after the next.

You will have noticed that the schemes for building simple cells from center-surround ones, as in the illustration on page 74, and for building complex cells out of simple ones, as in the illustration on this page, both involve excitatory processes. In the two cases, however, the processes must be very different. The first scheme requires *simultaneous* summed inputs from center-surround cells whose field centers lie along a line. In the second scheme, activation of the complex cell by a moving stimulus requires *successive* activation of many simple cells. It would be interesting to know what, if any, morphological differences underlie this difference in addition properties.

DIRECTIONAL SELECTIVITY

Many complex cells respond better to one direction of movement than to the diametrically opposite direction. The difference in response is often so marked that one direction of movement will produce a lively response and the other direction no response at all, as shown in the diagram on this page. It turns out that about 10 to 20 percent of cells in the upper layers of the striate cortex show marked directional selectivity. The rest seem not to care: we have to pay close attention or use a computer to see any difference in the responses to the two opposite directions. There seem to be two distinct classes of cells, one strongly direction-selective, the other not selective.

Listening to a strongly direction-selective cell respond, the feeling you get is that the line moving in one direction grabs the cell and pulls it along and that the line moving in the other direction fails utterly to engage it—something like the feeling you get with a ratchet, in winding a watch.

We don't know how such directionally selective cells are wired up. One possibility is that they are built up from simple cells whose responses to opposite directions of movement are asymmetric. Such simple cells have asymmetric fields, such as the one shown in the third diagram of the illustration on page 72. A second mechanism was proposed in 1965 by Horace Barlow and William Levick to explain the directional selectivity of certain cells in the rabbit retina—cells that apparently are not present in the monkey retina. If we apply their scheme to complex cells, we would suppose that interposed between simple and complex cells are intermediate cells, colored white in the diagram on the next page. We imagine that an intermediate cell receives excitation from one simple cell and inhibition from another (green) cell, whose receptive field is immediately adjacent and always located to one side and not the other. We

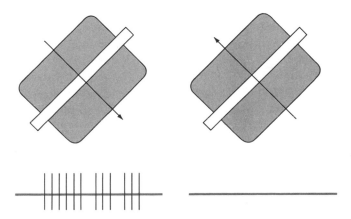

Responses of this complex cell differ to an optimally oriented slit moving in opposite directions. Each record is about 2 seconds in duration. (Cells such as this are not very fussy about how fast the slit moves; generally, responses fail only when the slit moves so fast that it becomes blurred or so slow that movement cannot be seen.)

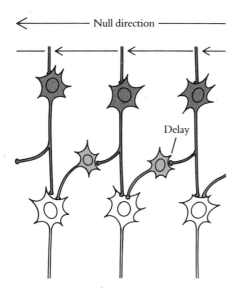

← —————— Null direction —————— →

Delay

Horace Barlow and William Levick proposed this circuit to explain directional selectivity. Synapses from purple to green are excitatory, and from green to white, inhibitory. We suppose the three white cells at the bottom converge on a single master cell.

further suppose that the inhibitory path involves a delay, perhaps produced by still another intermediate cell. Then, if the stimulus moves in one direction, say, right to left, as in the illustration of Barlow and Levick's model, the intermediate cell is excited by one of its inputs just as the inhibition arrives from the other, whose field has just been crossed. The two effects cancel, and the cell does not fire. For left-to-right movement, the inhibition arrives too late to prevent firing. If many such intermediate cells converge on a third cell, that cell will have the properties of a directionally selective complex cell.

We have little direct evidence for any schemes that try to explain the behavior of cells in terms of a hierarchy of complexity, in which cells at each successive level are constructed of building blocks from the previous level. Nevertheless, we have strong reasons for believing that the nervous system is organized in a hierarchical series. The strongest evidence is anatomical: for example, in the cat, simple cells are aggregated in the fourth layer of the striate cortex, the same layer that receives geniculate input, whereas the complex cells are located in the layers above and below, one or two synapses further along. Thus although we may not know the exact circuit diagram at each stage, we have good reasons to suppose the existence of some circuit.

The main reason for thinking that complex cells may be built up from center-surround cells, with a step in between, is the seeming necessity of doing the job in two logical steps. I should emphasize the word *logical* because the whole transformation presumably could be accomplished in one physical step by having center-surround inputs sum on separate dendritic branches of complex cells, with each branch doing the job of a simple cell, signaling electrotonically (by passive electrical spread) to the cell body, and hence to the axon, whenever a line falls in some particular part of the receptive field. The cell itself would then be complex. But the very existence of simple cells suggests that we do not have to imagine anything as complicated as this.

THE SIGNIFICANCE OF MOVEMENT-SENSITIVE CELLS, INCLUDING SOME COMMENTS ON HOW WE SEE

Why are movement-sensitive cells so common? An obvious first guess is that they tell us if the visual landscape contains a moving object. To animals, ourselves included, changes in the outside world are far more important than static conditions, for the survival of predator and prey alike. It is therefore no wonder that most cortical cells respond better to a moving object than to a stationary one. Having carried the logic this far, you may now begin to wonder how we analyze a stationary landscape at all if, in the interests of having high movement sensitivity, so many oriented cells are insensitive to stationary contours. The answer requires a short digression, which takes us to some basic, seemingly counterintuitive facts about how we see.

First, you might expect that in exploring our visual surroundings, we let our eyes freely rove around in smooth, continuous movement. What our two eyes in fact do is fixate on an object: we first adjust the positions of our eyes so that the images of the object fall on the two foveas; then we hold that position for a brief period, say, half a second; then our eyes suddenly jump to a new position by fixating on a new target whose presence somewhere out in the visual field has asserted itself, either by moving slightly, by contrasting with the background, or by presenting an interesting shape. During the jump, or *saccade,* which is French for "jolt", or "jerk" (the verb), the eyes move so rapidly that our visual system does not even respond to the resulting movement of the scene across the retina; we are altogether unaware of the violent change. (Vision may also in some sense be turned off during saccades by a complex circuit linking eye-movement centers with the visual path.) Exploring a visual scene, in reading or just looking around, is thus a process of having our eyes jump in rapid succession from one place to another.

Detailed monitoring of eye movements shows vividly how unaware we are of any of this. To monitor eye movements we first attach a tiny mirror to a contact lens, at the side, where it does not block vision; we then reflect a spot of light off the mirror onto a screen. Or, using a more modern version invented by David Robinson at the Wilmer Institute at Johns Hopkins, we can mount a tiny coil of wire around the rim of a contact lens, with the subject seated between two orthogonal pairs of bicycle-wheel size hoops containing coils of wire; currents in these coils induce currents in the contact-lens coil, which can be calibrated to give precise monitoring of eye movements. Neither method is what you would call a picnic for the poor subject.

In 1957, Russian psychophysicist A. L. Yarbus recorded eye movements of subjects as they explored various images, such as a woods or female faces (see the illustrations on the next page), by showing the stopping places of a subject's gaze as dots joined by lines indicating the eyes' trajectory during the jumps. A glance at these amazing pictures gives us a world of information about our vision—even about the objects and details that interest us in our environment.

So the first counterintuitive fact is that in visual exploration our eyes jump around from one point of interest to another: we cannot explore a stationary scene by swinging our eyes past it in continuous movements. The visual system seems intent instead on keeping the image of a scene anchored on our retinas, on preventing it from sliding around. If the whole scene moves by, as

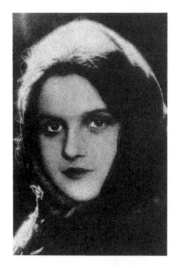

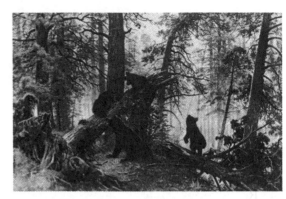

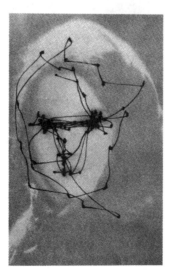

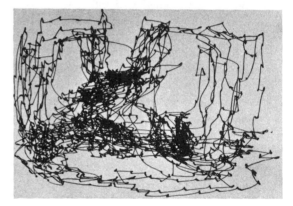

A picture is viewed by an observer while we monitor eye position and hence direction of gaze. The eyes jump, come to rest momentarily (producing a small dot on the record), then jump to a new locus of interest. It seems difficult to jump to a void—a place lacking abrupt luminance changes.

occurs when we look out a train window, we follow it by fixating on an object and maintaining fixation by moving our eyes until the object gets out of range, whereupon we make a saccade to a new object. This whole sequence—following with smooth pursuit, say, to the right, then making a saccade to the left—is called *nystagmus*. You can observe the sequence—perhaps next time you are in a moving train or streetcar—by looking at your neighbor's eyes as he or she looks out a window at the passing scene—taking care not to have your attentions misunderstood! The process of making visual saccades to items of interest, in order to get their images on the fovea, is carried out largely by the superior colliculus, as Peter Schiller at MIT showed in an impressive series of papers in the 1970s.

The second set of facts about how we see is even more counterintuitive. When we look at a stationary scene by fixating on some point of interest, our eyes lock onto that point, as just described, but the locking is not absolute. Despite any efforts we may make, the eyes do not hold perfectly still but make constant tiny movements called *microsaccades;* these occur several times per second and are more or less random in direction and about 1 to 2 minutes of arc in amplitude. In 1952 Lorrin Riggs and Floyd Ratliff, at Brown University, and R. W. Ditchburn and B. L. Ginsborg, at Reading University, simultaneously and independently found that if an image is optically artificially stabilized on the retina, eliminating any movement relative to the retina, vision fades away after about a second and the scene becomes quite blank! (The simplest way of stabilizing is to attach a tiny spotlight to a contact lens; as the eye moves, the spot moves too, and quickly fades.) Artificially moving the image on the retina, even by a tiny amount, causes the spot to reappear at once. Evidently, microsaccades are necessary for us to continue to see stationary objects. It is as if the visual system, after going to the trouble to make movement a powerful stimulus—wiring up cells so as to be insensitive to stationary objects—had then to invent microsaccades to make stationary objects visible.

We can guess that cortical complex cells, with their very high sensitivity to movement, are involved in this process. Directional selectivity is probably not involved, because microsaccadic movements are apparently random in direction. On the other hand, directional selectivity would seem very useful for detecting movements of objects against a stationary background, by telling us that a movement is taking place and in what direction. To follow a moving object against a stationary background, we have to lock onto the object and track it with our eyes; the rest of the scene then slips across the retina, an event that otherwise occurs only rarely. Such slippage, with every contour in the scene moving across the retina, must produce a tremendous storm of activity in our cortex.

END STOPPING

One additional kind of specificity occurs prominently in the striate cortex. An ordinary simple or complex cell usually shows length summation: the longer the stimulus line, the better is the response, until the line is as long as the receptive field; making the line still longer has no effect. For an *end-*

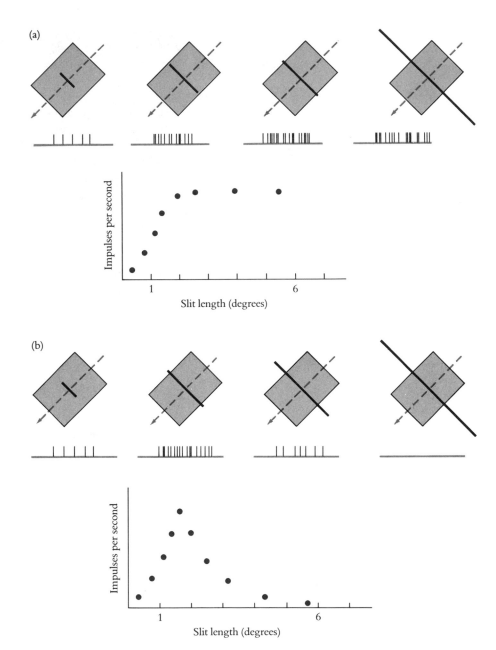

Top: An ordinary complex cell responds to various lengths of a slit of light. The duration of each record is 2 seconds. As indicated by the graph of response versus slit length, for this cell the response increases with length up to about 2 degrees, after which there is no change. *Bottom:* For this end-stopped cell, responses improve up to 2 degrees but then decline, so that a line 6 degrees or longer gives no response.

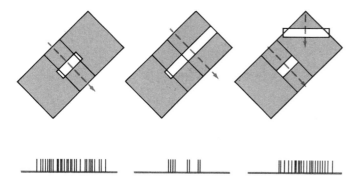

For this end-stopped cell, stimulating the middle activating region alone with an optimally oriented slit produces a strong response. Including one of the inhibitory regions almost nullifies the response, but if the inhibitory region is stimulated with a different orientation, the response is no longer blocked. Thus the activating region and the inhibitory regions both have the same optimal orientations.

stopped cell, lengthening the line improves the response up to some limit, but exceeding that limit in one or both directions results in a weaker response, as shown in the bottom diagram on the facing page. Some cells, which we call completely end stopped, do not respond at all to a long line. We call the region from which responses are evoked the *activating region* and speak of the regions at one or both ends as inhibitory. The total receptive field is consequently made up of the activating region and the inhibitory region or regions at the ends. The stimulus orientation that best evokes excitation in the activating region evokes maximal inhibition in the outlying area(s). This can be shown by repeatedly stimulating the activating region with an optimally oriented line of optimal length while testing the outlying region with lines of varying orientation, as shown in the top diagram on this page.

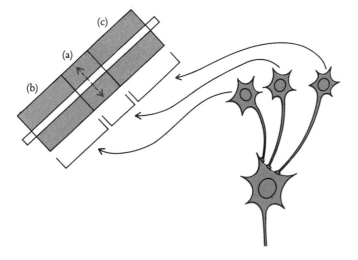

One scheme for explaining the behavior of a complex end-stopped cell. Three ordinary complex cells converge on the end-stopped cell: one, whose receptive field is congruent with the end-stopped cell's activating region (a), makes excitatory contacts; the other two, having fields in the outlying regions (b and c), make inhibitory contacts.

In an alternative scheme, one cell does the inhibiting, a cell whose receptive field covers the entire area (b). For this to work, we have to assume that the inhibiting cell responds only weakly to a short slit when (a) is stimulated, but responds strongly to a long slit.

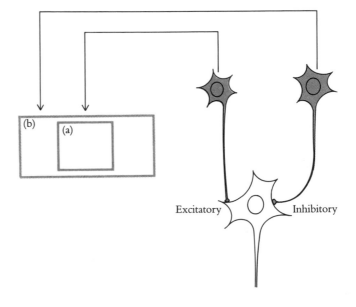

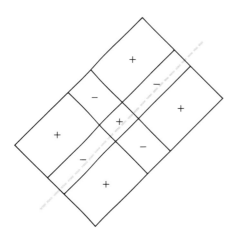

This end-stopped simple cell is assumed to result from convergent input from three ordinary simple cells. (One cell, with the middle on-center field, could excite the cell in question; the two others could be off center and also excite or be on center and inhibit.) Alternatively, the input to this cell could come directly from center-surround cells, by some more elaborate version of the process illustrated on page 74.

We originally thought that such cells represented a stage one step beyond complex cells in the hierarchy. In the simplest scheme for elaborating such a cell, the cell would be excited by one or a few ordinary complex cells with fields in the activating region and would be inhibited by complex cells with similarly oriented fields situated in the outlying regions. I have illustrated this scheme in the bottom diagram on the preceding page. A second possibility is that the cell receives excitatory input from cells with small fields, marked (a) in the diagram on this page, and inhibition from cells with large fields, marked (b); we assume that the cells supplying inhibition are maximally excited by long slits but poorly excited by short ones. This second possibility (analogous to the model for center-surround cells described on pages 52–53) is one of the few circuits for which we have some evidence. Charles Gilbert, at Rockefeller University in New York, has shown that complex cells in layer 6 of the monkey striate cortex have just the right properties for supplying this inhibition and, furthermore, that disabling these cells by local injections causes end-stopped cells in the upper layers to lose the end inhibition.

After these models were originally proposed, Geoffery Henry, in Canberra, Australia, discovered end-stopped simple cells, presumably with the receptive-field arrangement shown in the lower margin of this page. For such a cell, the wiring would be analogous to our first diagram, except that the input would be from simple rather than from complex cells. Complex end-stopped cells could thus arise by excitatory input from one set of complex cells and inhibitory input from another set, as in the diagrams on the two preceding pages, or by convergent input from many end-stopped simple cells.

The optimal stimulus for an end-stopped cell is a line that extends for a certain distance and no further. For a cell that responds to edges and is end stopped at one end only, a corner is ideal; for a cell that responds to slits or black bars and is stopped at both ends, the optimum stimulus is a short white or black line or a line that curves so that it is appropriate in the activating region and inappropriate—different by 20 to 30 degrees or more—in the flanking regions, as shown in the diagram of the curved contour on this page. We can thus view end-stopped cells as sensitive to corners, to curvature, or to sudden breaks in lines.

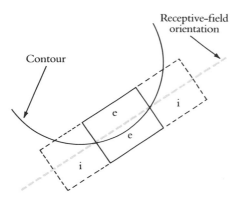

For an end-stopped cell such as the one shown on page 83, a curved border should be an effective stimulus.

THE IMPLICATIONS OF SINGLE-CELL PHYSIOLOGY FOR PERCEPTION

The fact that a cell in the brain responds to visual stimuli does not guarantee that it plays a direct part in perception. For example, many structures in the brainstem that are primarily visual have to do only with eye movements, pupillary constriction, or focusing by means of the lens. We can nevertheless be reasonably sure that the cells I described in this chapter have a lot to do with perception. As I mentioned at the outset, destroying any small piece of our striate cortex produces blindness in some small part of our visual world, and damaging the striate cortex has the same result in the monkey. In the cat things are not so simple: a cat with its striate cortex removed *can* see, though less well. Other parts of the brain, such as the superior colliculus, may play a relatively more important part in a cat's perception than they do in the primate's. Lower vertebrates, such as frogs and turtles, have nothing quite like our cortex, yet no one would contend that they are blind.

We can now say with some confidence what any one of these cortical cells is likely to be doing in response to a natural scene. The majority of cortical cells respond badly to diffuse light but well to appropriately oriented lines. Thus for the kidney shape shown in the illustration on the next page, such a cell will fire if and only if its receptive field is cut in the right orientation by the borders. Cells whose receptive fields are inside the borders will be unaffected; they will continue to fire at their spontaneous rate, oblivious to the presence or absence of the form.

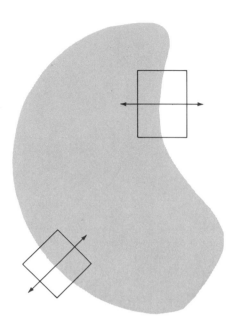

How are cells in our brain likely to respond to some everyday stimulus, such as this kidney-shaped uniform blob? In the visual cortex, only a select set of cells will show any interest.

This is the case for orientation-specific cells in general. But to evoke a response from a simple cell, a contour must do more than be oriented to match the optimum orientation of the cell; it must also fall in the simple cell's receptive field, almost exactly on a border between excitation and inhibition, because the excitatory part must be illuminated without encroachment on the inhibitory part. If we move the contour even slightly, without rotating it, it will no longer stimulate the cell; it will now activate an entirely new population of simple cells. For complex cells, conditions are much less stringent because whatever population of cells is activated by a stimulus at one instant will remain unchanged if the form is moved a small distance in any direction without rotation. To cause a marked change in the population of activated complex cells, a movement has to be large enough for the border to pass entirely out of the receptive fields of some complex cells and into the fields of others. Thus compared to the population of simple cells, the population of activated complex cells, as a whole, will not greatly change in response to small translational movements of an object.

Finally, for end-stopped cells, we similarly find an increased freedom in the exact placement of the stimulus, yet the population activated by any form will be far more select. For end-stopped cells, the contour's orientation must fit the cell's optimum orientation within the activating region but must differ enough just beyond the activating region so as not to annul the excitation. In short, the contour must be curved just enough to fit the cell's requirements, or it must terminate abruptly, as shown in the diagram of the curve (page 85).

One result of these exacting requirements is to increase efficiency, in that an object in the visual field stimulates only a tiny fraction of the cells on whose receptive fields it falls. The increasing cell specialization underlying this efficiency is likely to continue as we go further and deeper into the central nervous system, beyond the striate cortex. Rods and cones are influenced by light as such. Ganglion cells, geniculate cells, and center-surround cortical cells compare a region with its surrounds and are therefore likely to be influenced by any contours that cut their receptive fields but will not be influenced by overall changes in light intensity. Orientation-specific cells care not only about the presence of a contour but also about its orientation and even its rate of change of orientation—its curvature. When such cells are complex, they are also sensitive to movement. We can see from the discussion in the last section that movement sensitivity can have two interpretations: it could help draw attention to moving objects, or it could work in conjunction with microsaccades to keep complex cells firing in response to stationary objects.

I suspect light-dark contours are the most important component of our perception, but they are surely not the only component. The coloring of objects certainly helps in defining their contours, although our recent work tends to emphasize the limitations of color in defining forms. The shading of objects, consisting of gradual light-dark transitions, as well as their textures, can give important clues concerning shape and depth. Although the cells we have been discussing could conceivably contribute to the perception of shading and texture, we would certainly not expect them to respond to either quality with enthusiasm. How our brain handles textures is still not clear. One guess is that complex cells do mediate shades and textures without the help of any other specialized sets of cells. Such stimuli may not activate many cells very efficiently, but the spatial extension that is an essential attribute of shading or texture may make many cells respond, all in a moderate or weak way. Perhaps lukewarm responses from many cells are enough to transmit the information to higher levels.

Many people, including myself, still have trouble accepting the idea that the interior of a form (such as the kidney bean on the facing page) does not itself excite cells in our brain—that our awareness of the interior as black or white (or colored, as we will see in Chapter 8) depends only on cells sensitive to the borders. The intellectual argument is that the perception of an evenly lit interior depends on the activation of cells having fields at the borders and on the absence of activation of cells whose fields are within the borders, since such activation would indicate that the interior is not evenly lit. So our perception of the interior as black, white, gray, or green has nothing to do with cells whose fields are in the interior—hard as that may be to swallow. But if an engineer were designing a machine to encode such a form, I think this is exactly what he would do. What happens at the borders is the only information you need to know: the interior is boring. Who could imagine that the brain would not evolve in such a way as to handle the information with the least number of cells?

After hearing about simple and complex cells, people often complain that the analysis of every tiny part of our visual field—for all possible orientations and for dark lines, light lines, and edges—must surely require an astronomic number of cells. The answer is yes, certainly. But that fits perfectly, because an astronomic number of cells is just what the cortex has. Today we can say what the cells in this part of the brain are doing, at least in response to many simple, everyday visual stimuli. I suspect that no two striate cortical cells do exactly the same thing, because whenever a microelectrode tip succeeds in recording from two cells at a time, the two show slight differences—in exact receptive field position, directional selectivity, strength of response, or some other attribute. In short, there seems to be little redundancy in this part of the brain.

How sure can we be that these cells are not wired up to respond to some other stimulus besides straight line segments? It is not as though we and others have not tried many other stimuli, including faces, Cosmopolitan covers, and waving our hands. Experience shows that we would be foolish to think that we had exhausted the list of possibilities. In the early 1960s, just when we felt satisfied with the striate cortex and wanted to move on to the next area (in fact, we *had* moved on), we happened to record from a sluggishly responding cell in the striate cortex and, by making the slit shorter, found that this very cell was anything but a sluggish responder. In this way we stumbled on end stopping. And it took almost twenty years work with the monkey striate cortex before we became aware of blobs—pockets of cells specialized for color, described in Chapter 8. Having expressed these reservations, I should add that I have no doubt at all that some of the findings, such as orientation selectivity, are genuine properties of these cells. There is too much collateral evidence, such as the functional anatomy, described in Chapter 5, to allow for much scepticism.

BINOCULAR CONVERGENCE

I have so far made little mention of the existence of two eyes. Obviously, we need to ask whether any cortical cells receive input from both eyes and, if so, whether the two inputs are generally equal, qualitatively or quantitatively.

To get at these questions we have to backtrack for a moment to the lateral geniculate body and ask if any of the cells there can be influenced from both eyes. The lateral geniculate body represents the first opportunity for information from the two eyes to come together at the level of the single cell. But it seems that the opportunity there is missed: the two sets of input are consigned to separate sets of layers, with little or no opportunity to combine. As we would expect from this segregation, a geniculate cell responds to one eye and not at all to the other. Some experiments have indicated that stimuli to the otherwise ineffective eye can subtly influence responses from the first eye. But for all practical purposes, each cell seems to be virtually monopolized by one or the other eye.

Intuitively, it would seem that the paths from the two eyes must sooner or later converge, because when we look at a scene we see one unified picture. It is nevertheless everyone's experience that covering one eye makes no great difference in what we see: things seem about as clear, as vivid, and as bright. We see a bit farther to the side with both eyes, of course, because the retinas do not extend around as far in an outward (temporal) direction as they extend inwardly (nasally); still, the difference is only about 20 to 30 degrees. (Remember that the visual environment is inverted and reversed on the retina by the optics of the eye.) The big difference between one-eyed and two-eyed vision is in the sense of depth, a subject taken up in Chapter 7.

In the monkey cortex, the cells that receive the input from the geniculates, those whose fields have circular symmetry, are also like geniculate cells in being monocular. We find about an equal number of left-eye and right-eye cells, at least in parts of the cortex subserving vision up to about 20 degrees from the direction of gaze. Beyond this center-surround stage, however, we find binocular cells, simple and complex. In the macaque monkey over half of these higher-order cells can be influenced independently from the two eyes.

Once we have found a binocular cell we can compare in detail the receptive fields in the two eyes. We first cover the right eye and map the cell's receptive field in the left eye, noting its exact position on the screen or retina and its complexity, orientation, and arrangement of excitatory and inhibitory regions; we ask if the cell is simple or complex, and we look for end stopping and directional selectivity. Now we block off the left eye and uncover the right, repeating all the questions. In most binocular cells, we find that all the properties found in the left eye hold also for the right-eye stimulation—the same position in the visual field, the same directional selectivity, and so on. So we can say that the connections or circuits between the left eye and the cell we are studying are present as a duplicate copy between the right eye and that cell.

We need to make one qualification concerning this duplication of connections. If, having found the best stimulus—orientation, position, movement

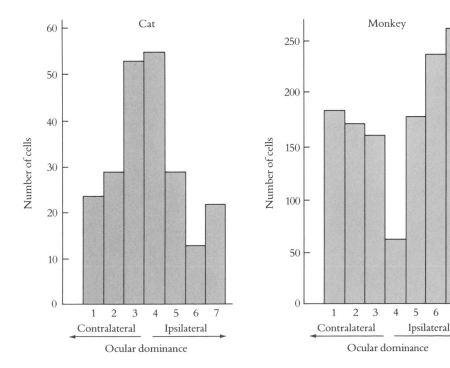

In population studies of ocular dominance, we study hundreds of cells and categorize each one as belonging to one of seven arbitrary groups. A group 1 cell is defined as a cell influenced only by the contralateral eye—the eye opposite to the hemisphere in which it sits. A group 2 cell responds to both eyes but strongly prefers the contralateral eye. And so on.

direction, and so on—we then compare the responses evoked from one eye with the responses evoked from the other, we find that the two responses are not necessarily equally vigorous. Some cells do respond equally to the two eyes, but others consistently give a more powerful discharge to one eye than to the other. Overall, except for the part of the cortex subserving parts of the visual field well away from the direction of gaze, we find no obvious favoritism: in a given hemisphere, just as many cells favor the eye on the opposite side (the *contralateral* eye) as the eye on the same side (the *ipsilateral*). All shades of relative eye dominance are represented, from cells monopolized by the left eye through cells equally affected to cells responding only to the right eye.

We can now do a population study. We group all the cells we have studied, say 1000 of them, into seven arbitrary groups, according to the relative effectiveness of the two eyes; we then compare their numbers, as shown in the two bar graphs on the preceding page. At a glance the histograms tell us how the distribution differs between cat and monkey: that in both species, binocular cells are common, with each eye well represented (roughly equally, in the monkey); that in cats, binocular cells are very abundant; that in macaques, monocular and binocular cells are about equally common, but that binocular cells often favor one eye strongly (groups 2 and 5).

We can go even further and ask if binocular cells respond better to both eyes than to one. Many do: separate eyes may do little or nothing, but both together produce a strong discharge, especially when the two eyes are stimulated simultaneously in exactly the same way. The figure on this page shows a recording from three cells (1, 2, and 3), all of which show strong synergy. One

The recording electrode was close enough to three cells to pick up impulses from all of them. Responses could be distinguished by size and shape of the impulses. This illustrates the responses to stimuli to single eyes and to both eyes. Cells (1) and (2) both would be in group 4 since they responded about equally to the two eyes. Cell (3) responded only when both eyes were stimulated; we can say only that it was not a group 1 or a group 7 cell.

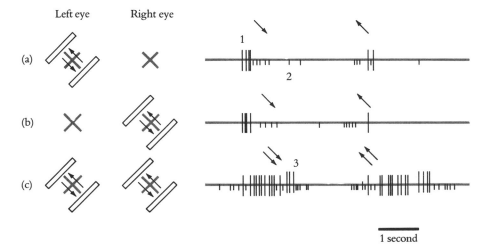

Left eye   Right eye

(a)

(b)

(c)

1 second

of the three did not respond at all to either eye alone, and thus its presence would have gone undetected had we not stimulated the two eyes together. Many cells show little or no synergistic effect; they respond about the same way to both eyes together as to either eye alone.

A special class of binocular cells, wired up so as to respond specifically to near or far objects, will be taken up separately when we come to discuss stereopsis, in Chapter 7.

These hookups from single cells to the two eyes illustrate once more the high degree of specificity of connections in the brain. As if it were not remarkable enough that a cell can be so connected as to respond to only one line orientation and one movement direction, we now learn that the connections are laid down in duplicate copies, one from each eye. And as if that were not remarkable enough, most of the connections, as we will see in Chapter 9, seem to be wired up and ready to go at birth.

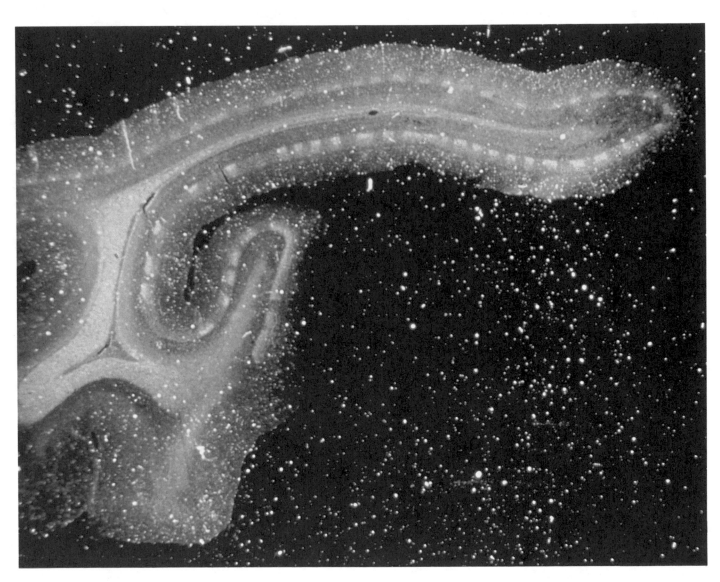

Ocular-dominance columns are seen in this section through a macaque monkey's left striate cortex, taken perpendicular to the surface in a left-to-right direction. As we follow the part of the cortex that is exposed to the surface from left to right (top of photo), it bends around forming a buried fold that extends from right to left. Radioactive amino acid injected into the left eye has been transported through the lateral geniculate body to layer 4C, where it occupies a series of half-millimeter-wide patches; these glow brightly in this dark-field picture. (The continuous leaflet in the middle is white matter, containing the geniculo-cortical fibers.)

5

THE ARCHITECTURE
OF THE VISUAL CORTEX

The primary visual, or striate, cortex is a far more complex and elaborate structure than either the lateral geniculate body or the retina. We have already seen that the sudden increase in structural complexity is accompanied by a dramatic increase in physiological complexity. In the cortex we find a greater variety of physiologically defined cell types, and the cells respond to more elaborate stimuli, especially to a greater number of stimulus parameters that have to be properly specified. We are concerned not only with stimulus position and spot size, as we are in the retina and geniculate, but now suddenly with line orientation, eye dominance, movement direction, line length, and curvature. What if anything is the relation between these variables and the structural organization of the cortex? To address this question, I will need to begin by saying something about the structure of the striate cortex.

ANATOMY OF THE VISUAL CORTEX

The cerebral cortex, which almost entirely covers the cerebral hemispheres, has the general form of a plate whose thickness is about 2 millimeters and whose surface area in humans is over 1 square foot. The total area of the macaque monkey's cortex is much less, probably about one-tenth that of the human. We have known for over a century that this plate is subdivided into a patchwork of many different *cortical areas;* of these, the primary visual cortex was the first to be distinguished from the rest by its layered or striped appearance in cross section—hence its classical name, striate cortex. At one time the entire careers of neuroanatomists consisted of separating off large numbers of cortical areas on the basis of sometimes subtle histological distinctions, and in one popular numbering system the striate cortex was assigned the

A large part of the cerebral cortex on the right side has been exposed under local anesthesia for the neurosurgical treatment of seizures in this fully conscious human patient. The surgeon was Dr. William Feindel at the Montreal Neurological Institute. The scalp has been opened and retracted and a large piece of skull removed. (It is replaced at the end of the operation.) You can see gyri and sulci, and the large purplish veins and smaller, red, less conspicuous arteries. The overall pinkish appearance is caused by the finer branches of these vessels. Filling the bottom third of the exposure is the temporal lobe; above the prominent, horizontally running veins are the parietal lobe, to the left, and frontal lobe, to the right. At the extreme left we see part of the occipital lobe. This operation, for the treatment of a particular type of epilepsy, consists of removing diseased brain, which is only permissible if it does not result in impairment of voluntary movement or loss of speech. To avoid this, the neurosurgeon identifies speech, motor, and sensory areas by electrical stimulation, looking for movements, sensations related precisely to different parts of the body, or interference with speech. Such tests would obviously not be possible if the patient were not conscious. Points that have been stimulated have been labeled by the tiny numbered sterile patches of paper. For example, stimulation of these regions gave the following results: (1) tingling sensation in the left thumb; (2) tingling in the left ring finger; (3) tingling in the left middle and ring finger; (4) flexion of left fingers and wrist. The regions labeled 8 and 13 gave more complex memory-like sensations typically produced on stimulation of the temporal lobe in certain types of epileptic patients.

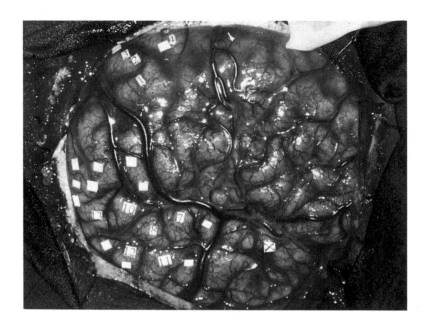

number 17. According to one of the more recent estimates by David Van Essen of Caltech, the macaque monkey primary visual cortex occupies 1200 square millimeters—a little less than one-third the area of a credit card. This represents about 15 percent of the total cortical area in the macaque, certainly a substantial fraction of the entire cortex.

A rear view of the brain of a macaque monkey is seen in the photograph on the next page. The skull has been removed and the brain perfused for preservation with a dilute solution of formaldehyde, which colors it yellow. Blood vessels normally form a conspicuous web over the surface, but here they are collapsed and not visible. What we see in this rear view is mostly the surface of the occipital lobe of the cortex, the area that is concerned with vision and that comprises not only the striate cortex but also one or two dozen or more *prestriate* areas. To get a half-millimeter-thick plate of nervous tissue that is the area of a large index card into a box the size of the monkey's skull necessitates some folding and crinkling, the way you crinkle up a piece of paper before throwing it into the waste basket; this produces fissures, or *sulci*, between which are ridges, or *gyri*.

The area behind (below, in this photograph) the dotted line is the exposed part of the striate cortex. Although the striate cortex occupies most of the surface of the occipital lobe, we can see only about one-third to one-half of it in the photograph; the rest is hidden out of sight in a fissure.

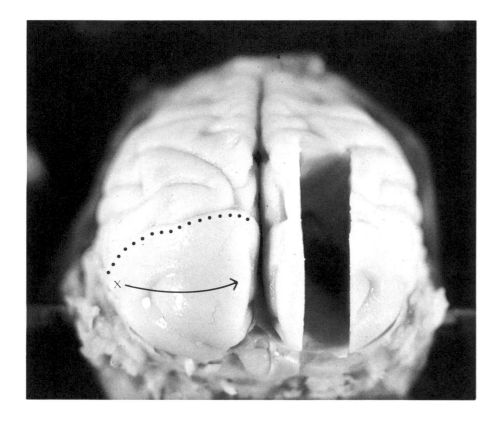

This view of a macaque monkey's brain, from behind, shows the occipital lobe and the part of the striate cortex visible on the surface (below the dotted line).

The striate cortex (area 17) sends much of its output to the next cortical region, *visual area 2,* also called *area 18* because it is next door to area 17. Area 18 forms a band of cortex about 6 to 8 millimeters wide, which almost completely surrounds area 17. We can just see part of area 18 in the photograph, above the dotted line, the boundary between 17 and 18, but most of it extends down into the deep sulcus just in front of that line. Area 17 projects to area 18 in a plate-to-plate, orderly fashion. Area 18 in turn projects to at least three postage-stamp-size occipital regions, called MT (for medial temporal), visual area 3, and visual area 4 (often abbreviated V3 and V4). And so it goes, with each area projecting forward to several other areas. In addition, each of these areas projects back to the area or areas from which it receives input. As if that were not complicated enough, each of the areas projects to structures deep in the brain, for example to the superior colliculus and to various subdivisions of the thalamus (a complex golf-ball-size mass of cells, of which the lateral geniculate forms a small part). And each of these visual areas receives input from a thalamic subdivision: just as the geniculate projects to the primary visual cortex, so other parts project to the other areas.

In the same photograph, X indicates the part of area 17 that receives information from the foveas, or centers of gaze, of the two retinas. As we move from X, in the left hemisphere, toward the arrowhead, the corresponding point in the right half of the visual field starts in the center of gaze and moves out, to the right, along the horizon. Starting again from X, movement to the right along the border between areas 17 and 18 corresponds to movement down in the visual field; movement back corresponds to movement up. The arrowhead marks a region about 6 degrees out along the horizon. The visual field farther out than 9 degrees is represented on the part of area 17 that is folded underneath the surface and parallel to it.

To see what the cortex looks like in cross section, we have cut a chunk from the visual cortex on the right side of the photograph on page 95. The resulting cross section, as in the photomicrograph on this page, is stained with cresyl violet, a dye that colors the cell bodies dark blue but does not stain axons or dendrites. With the photomicrograph taken at this low power, we cannot distinguish individual cells, but we can see dark layers of densely aggregated cells and lighter layers of more thinly scattered ones. Beneath the exposed part of the cortex, we see a mushroom-shaped, buried part that is folded under in a complicated way, but these two parts are actually continuous. The lightly stained substance is white matter; it lies under the part of the cortex that is

This cross section through the occipital lobe was made by cutting out a piece as shown in the photograph on page 95. It is what we would see if we were to walk into the groove and look to the left. The letter *a* corresponds to a point halfway between X and the arrowhead. The Nissl stain shows cell bodies only; these are too small to make out except as dots. The darker part of the top and the mushroom-shaped part just below are striate cortex. The three letter *d*'s mark the border between areas 17 and 18.

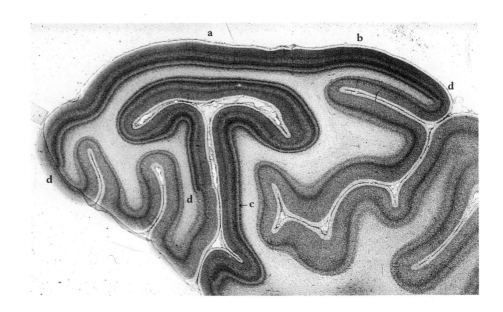

exposed to the surface, separating it from the buried fold of cortex, and consists mainly of myelinated nerve fibers, which do not stain. The cortex, containing nerve-cell bodies, axons, dendrites, and synapses, is an example of gray matter.

For anatomical richness, in its complexity of layering, area 17 exceeds every other part of the cortex. You can see an indication of this complexity even in this low-magnification cross section when you compare area 17 with its next-door neighbor, area 18, bordering area 17 at *d*. What is more, as we look along the cross section from the region marked *a*, which is a few degrees from the foveal projection to the cortex, toward the region marked *b*, 6 degrees out, or toward *c,* 80 to 90 degrees out, we see very little change in the thickness or the layering pattern. This uniformity turns out to be important, and I will return to it in Chapter 6.

LAYERS OF THE VISUAL CORTEX

A small length of area 17 appears at higher magnification in the photomicrograph on this page. We can now make out the individual cell bodies as dots and get some idea of their size, numbers, and spacing. The layering

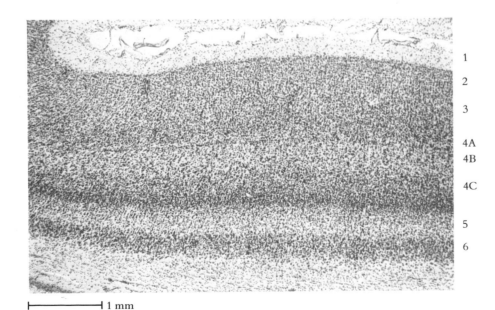

1
2
3
4A
4B
4C
5
6

⊢————⊣ 1 mm

A cross section of the striate cortex taken at higher magnification shows cells arranged in layers. Layers 2 and 3 are indistinguishable; layer 4A is very thin. The thick, light layer at the bottom is white matter.

pattern here is partly the result of variations in the staining and packing density of these cells. Layers 4C and 6 are densest and darkest; layers 1, 4B, and 5 are most loosely packed. Layer 1 contains hardly any nerve cells but has abundant axons, dendrites, and synapses. To show that different layers contain different kinds of cells requires a stain like that devised by Camillo Golgi in 1900. The Golgi stain reveals only occasional cells, but when it does reveal a cell, it may show it completely, including its axons and dendrites. The two major classes of cortical cells are the pyramidal cells, which occur in all layers except 1 and 4, and the stellate cells, which are found in all layers. You have seen an example of a pyramidal cell and a stellate cell in Chapter 1 (page 6). We can get a better idea of the distribution of pyramidal cells within the cortex in another drawing from Ramón y Cajal's *Histologie* (on this page), which shows perhaps 1 percent of pyramds instead of only one or two cells.

The fibers coming to the cortex from the lateral geniculate body enter from the white matter. Running diagonally, most make their way up to layer 4C, branching again and again, and finally terminate by making synapses with the stellate cells that populate that layer. Axons originating from the two ventral (magnocellular) geniculate layers end in the upper half of 4C, called 4Cα; those

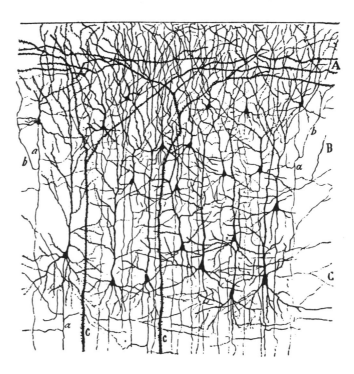

A Golgi-stained section from the upper layers, 1, 2, and 3, of the visual cortex in a child several days old. Black triangular dots are cell bodies, from which emanate an apical dendrite ascending and dividing in layer 1, basal dendrites coming off laterally, and a single slender axon heading straight down.

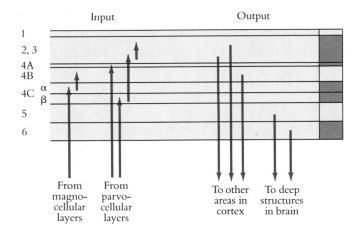

The main connections made by axons from the lateral geniculate body to the striate cortex and from the striate cortex to other brain regions. To the right, the shading indicates the relative density of Nissl staining, for comparison with the illustration on page 97.

from the four dorsal (parvocellular) geniculate layers end in the lower half of 4C (4Cβ). As you can see from the diagram on this page, these subdivisions of layer 4C have different projections to the upper layers: 4Cα sends its output to 4B; 4Cβ, to the deepest part of 3. And those layers in turn differ in their projections. Seeing these differences in the pathways stemming from the two sets of geniculate layers is one of many reasons to think that they represent two different systems. Most pyramidal cells in layers 2, 3, 4A, 5, and 6 send axons out of the cortex, but side-branches, called "collaterals", of these same descending axons connect locally and help to distribute the information through the full cortical thickness.

The layers of the cortex differ not only in their inputs and their local interconnections but also in the more distant structures to which they project. All layers except 1, 4A, and 4C send fibers out of the cortex. Layers 2 and 3 and layer 4B project mainly to other cortical regions, whereas the deep layers project down to subcortical structures: layer 5 projects to the superior colliculus in the midbrain, and layer 6 projects mainly back to the lateral geniculate body. Although we have known for almost a century that the inputs from the geniculate go mostly to layer 4, we did not know the differences in outputs of the different cortical layers until 1969, when Japanese scientist Keisuke Toyama first discovered them with physiological techniques; they have been confirmed anatomically many times since.

Ramón y Cajal was the first to realize how short the connections within the cortex are. As already described, the richest connections run up and down, intimately linking the different layers. Diagonal and side-to-side connections generally run for 1 or 2 millimeters, although a few travel up to 4 or 5 millimeters. This limitation in lateral spread of information has profound consequences. If the inputs are topographically organized—in the case of the visual system, organized according to retinal or visual-field position—the same must be true for the outputs. Whatever the cortex is doing, the analysis must be local. Information concerning some small part of the visual world comes in to a small piece of the cortex, is transformed, analyzed, digested—whatever expression you find appropriate—and is sent on for further processing somewhere else, without reference to what goes on next door. The visual scene is thus analyzed piecemeal. The primary visual cortex cannot therefore be the part of the brain where whole objects—boats, hats, faces—are recognized, perceived, or otherwise handled; it cannot be where "perception" resides. Of course, such a sweeping conclusion would hardly be warranted from anatomy alone. It could be that information is transmitted along the cortex for long distances in bucket-brigade fashion, spreading laterally in steps of 1 millimeter or so. We can show that this is not the case by recording while stimulating the retina: all the cells in a given small locality have small receptive fields, and any cell and its neighbor always have their receptive fields in very nearly the same place in the retina. Nothing in the physiology suggests that any cell in the monkey primary visual cortex talks to any other cell more than 2 or 3 millimeters away.

For centuries, similar hints had come from clinical neurology. A small stroke, tumor, or injury to part of the primary visual cortex can lead to blindness in a small, precisely demarcated island in the visual field; we find perfectly normal vision elsewhere, instead of the overall mild reduction in vision that we might expect if each cell communicated in some measure with all other cells. To digress slightly, we can note here that such a stroke patient may be unaware of anything wrong, especially if the defect is not in the foveal representation of the cortex and hence in the center of gaze—at least he will not perceive in his visual field an island of blackness or greyness or indeed anything at all. Even if the injury has destroyed one entire occipital lobe, leaving the subject blind in the entire half visual field on the other side, the result is not any active sensation of the world being blotted out on that side. My occasional migraine attacks (luckily without the headache) produce transient blindness, often in a large part of one visual field; if asked *what* I see there, I can only say, literally, nothing—not white, grey, or black, but just what I see directly behind—nothing.

Another curious feature of an island of localized blindness, or *scotoma*, is known as "completion". When someone with a scotoma looks at a line that passes through his blind region, he sees no interruption: the line is perfectly continuous. You can demonstrate the same thing using your own eye and blind spot, which you can find with no more apparatus than a cotton Q-tip. The blind spot is the region where the optic nerve enters the eye, an oval about 2 millimeters in diameter, with no rods and cones. The procedure for mapping it is so childishly simple that anyone who hasn't should! You start by closing one eye, say the left; keeping it closed, you fix your gaze with the other eye on a small object across the room. Now hold the Q-tip at arm's length directly in front of the object and slowly move it out to the right exactly horizontally (a dark background helps). The white cotton will vanish when it is about 18 degrees out. Now, if you place the stick so that it runs through the blind spot, it will still appear as a single stick, without any gap. The region of blindness constituting the blind spot is like any scotoma; you are not aware of it and cannot be, unless you test for it. You don't see black or white or anything there, you see nothing.

In an analogous way, if looking at a big patch of white paper activates only cells whose fields are cut by the paper's borders (since a cortical cell tends to ignore diffuse change in light), then the death of cells whose fields are within the patch of paper should make no difference. The island of blindness should not be seen—and it isn't. We don't see our blind spot as a black hole when we look at a big patch of white. The completion phenomenon, plus looking at a big white screen and verifying that there is no black hole where the optic disc is, should convince anyone that the brain works in ways that we cannot easily predict using intuition alone.

ARCHITECTURE OF THE CORTEX

Now we can return to our initial question: How are the physiological properties of cortical cells related to their structural organization? We can sharpen the question by restating it: Knowing that cells in the cortex can differ in receptive-field position, complexity, orientation preference, eye dominance, optimal movement direction, and best line length, should we expect neighboring cells to be similar in any or all of these, or could cells with different properties simply be peppered throughout the cortex at random, without regard to their physiological attributes?

Just looking at the anatomy with the unaided eye or under the microscope is of little help. We see clear variations in a cross section through the cortex from one layer to the next, but if we run our eye along any one layer or examine the cortex under a microscope in a section cut parallel to the layers, we see only a gray uniformity. Although that uniformity might seem to argue for randomness, we already know that for at least one variable, cells are distributed with a high degree of order. The fact that visual fields are mapped systematically onto the striate cortex tells us at once that neighboring cells in the cortex will have receptive fields close to each other in the visual fields. Experimentally that is exactly what we find. Two cells sitting side by side in the cortex invariably have their fields close together, and usually they overlap over most of their extent. They are nevertheless hardly ever precisely superimposed. As the electrode moves along the cortex from cell to cell, the receptive-field positions gradually change in a direction predicted from the known topographic map. No one would have doubted this result even fifty years ago, given what was known about geniculo-cortical connections and about the localized blindness resulting from strokes. But what about eye dominance, complexity, orientation, and all the other variables?

It took a few years to learn how to stimulate and record from cortical cells reliably enough to permit questions not just about individual cells but about large groups of cells. A start came when, by chance, we occasionally recorded from two or more cells at the same time. You already saw an example of this on page 90. To record from two neighboring cells is not difficult. In experiments where we ask about the stimulus preferences of cells, we almost always employ extracellular recording, placing the electrode tip just outside the cell and sampling currents associated with impulses rather than the voltage across the membrane. We frequently find ourselves recording from more than one cell at a time, say by having the electrode tip halfway between two cell bodies. Impulses from any single cell in such a record are all almost identical, but the size and shape of the spikes is affected by distance and geometry, so that impulses from two cells recorded at the same time are usually different and hence easily distinguished. With such a two-cell recording we can vividly demonstrate both how neighboring cells differ and what they can have in common.

One of the first two-unit recordings made from visual cortex showed two cells responding to opposite directions of movement of a hand waving back and forth in front of the animal. In that case, two cells positioned side by side in the cortex had different, in fact opposite, behaviors with respect to movement. In other respects, however, they almost certainly had similar properties. Had I known enough to examine their orientation preferences in 1956, I would very likely have found that both orientation preferences were close to vertical, since the cells responded so well to horizontal movements. The fact that they both responded when the moving hand crossed back and forth over the same region in space means that their receptive-field positions were about the same. Had I tested for eye dominance, I would likely have found it also to be the same for the two cells.

Even in the earliest cortical recordings, we were struck by how often the two cells in a two-unit recording had the same ocular dominance, the same complexity, and most striking of all, exactly the same orientation preference. Such occurrences, which could hardly be by chance, immediately suggested that cells with common properties were aggregated together. The possibility of such groupings was intriguing, and once we had established them as a reality, we began a search to learn more about their size and shape.

EXPLORATION OF THE CORTEX

Microelectrodes are one-dimensional tools. To explore a three-dimensional structure in the brain, we push an electrode slowly forward, stop at intervals to record from and examine a cell, or perhaps two or three cells, note the depth reading of the advancer, and then go on. Sooner or later the electrode tip penetrates all the way through the cortex. We can then pull the electrode out and reinsert it somewhere else. After the experiment, we slice, stain, and examine the tissue to determine the position of every cell that was recorded. In a single experiment, lasting about 24 hours, it is usual to make two or three electrode penetrations through the cortex, each about 4 to 5 millimeters long, and from each of which some 200 cells can be observed.

The electrodes are slender, and we do well if we can even find their tracks under a microscope; we consequently have no reason to think that in a long penetration enough cells are injured to impair measurably the responses of nearby cells. Originally it was hard to find the electrode track histologically, to say nothing of estimating the final position of the electrode tip, and it was consequently hard to estimate the positions of the cells that had been recorded. The problem was solved when it was discovered that by passing a tiny current through the electrode we could destroy cells in a small sphere centered on the electrode tip and could easily see this region of destruction histologically. Luckily, passing the current did no damage to the electrode, so that by making three or four such lesions along a single penetration and noting their depth readings and the depth readings of the recorded cells, we could estimate the position of each cell. The lesions, of course, kill a few cells near the electrode tip, but not enough to impair responses of cells a short distance away. For cells beyond the electrode tip, we can avoid losing information by going ahead a bit and recording before pulling back to make the lesion.

VARIATIONS IN COMPLEXITY

As we would expect, cells near the input end of the cortex, in layer 4, show less complicated behavior than cells near the output. In the monkey, as noted in this chapter, cells in layer $4C\beta$, which receive input from the upper four (parvocellular) geniculate layers, all seem to have center-surround properties, without orientation selectivity. In layer $4C\alpha$, whose input is from the ventral (magnocellular) pair of geniculate layers, some cells have center-surround fields, but others seem to be orientation-specific, with simple receptive fields. Farther downstream, in the layers above and below 4C, the great majority of cells are complex. End-stopping occurs in about 20 percent of cells in layers 2 and 3 but seldom occurs elsewhere. On the whole, then, we find a

A rough indication of physiological cell types found in the different layers of the striate cortex.

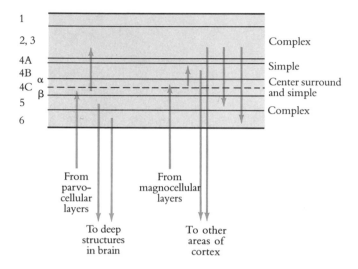

loose correlation between complexity and distance along the visual path, measured in numbers of synapses.

Stating that most cells above and below layer 4 are complex glosses over major layer-to-layer differences, because complex cells are far from all alike. They all have in common the defining characteristic of complex cells—they respond throughout their receptive field to a properly oriented moving line regardless of its exact position—but they differ in other ways. We can distinguish four subtypes that tend to be housed in different layers. In layers 2 and 3, most complex cells respond progressively better the longer the slit (they show *length summation*), and the response becomes weaker when the line exceeds a critical length only if a cell is end stopped. For cells in layer 5, short slits, covering only a small part of the length of a receptive field, work about as well as long ones; the receptive fields are much larger than the fields of cells in layers 2 and 3. For cells in layer 6, in contrast, the longer an optimally oriented line is, the stronger are the responses, until the line spans the entire length of the field, which is several times greater than the width (the distance over which a moving line evokes responses). The field is thus long and narrow. We can conclude that axons running from layers 5, 6, and 2 and 3 to different targets in the brain (the superior culliculus, geniculate, the other visual cortical areas) must carry somewhat different kinds of visual information.

In summary, from layer to layer we find differences in the way cells behave that seem more fundamental than differences, say, in optimal orientation or in ocular dominance. The most obvious of these layer-to-layer differences is in response complexity, which reflects the simple anatomical fact that some layers are closer than others to the input.

OCULAR-DOMINANCE COLUMNS

Eye-dominance groupings of cells in the striate cortex were the first to be recognized, largely because they are rather coarse. Because we now have many methods for examining them, they are now the best-known subdivision. It was obvious soon after the first recordings from monkeys that every time the electrode entered the cortex perpendicular to the surface, cell after cell favored the same eye, as shown in the illustration on this page. If the electrode was pulled out and reinserted at a new site a few millimeters away, one eye would again dominate, perhaps the same eye and perhaps the other one. In layer 4C, which receives the input from the geniculates, the dominant eye seemed to have not merely an advantage, but a monopoly. In the layers above and below, and hence farther along in the succession of synapses, over half of the cells could also be influenced from the nondominant eye—we call these cells *binocular*.

If instead of placing the electrode perpendicular to the surface, we introduced it obliquely, as close to parallel to the surface as could be managed, the eye dominance alternated back and forth, now one eye dominating and now the other. A complete cycle, from one eye to the other and back, occurred roughly once every millimeter. Obviously, the cortex seen from above must consist of some kind of mosaic composed of left-eye and right-eye regions.

The basis of the eye alternation became clear when new staining methods revealed how single geniculo-cortical axons branch and distribute themselves in the cortex. The branches of a single axon are such that its thousands of terminals form two or three clumps in layer 4C, each 0.5 millimeter wide,

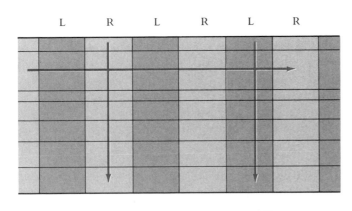

L   R   L   R   L   R

1 millimeter

Ocular dominance remains constant in vertical microelectrode penetrations through the striate cortex. Penetrations parallel to the surface show alternation from left eye to right eye and back, roughly one cycle every millimeter.

Each geniculate axon ascends through the deep layers of the striate cortex, subdividing repeatedly, finally terminating in 4C in 0.5 millimeter-wide clusters of synaptic endings, separated by blank areas, also 0.5 millimeter wide. All fibers from one eye occupy the same patches: the gaps are occupied by the other eye. The horizontal extent of the patches from a single fiber may be 2 to 3 millimeters for magnocellular terminals in 4Cα; a parvocellular fiber branches in a more restricted area in 4Cβ and generally occupies only one or two patches.

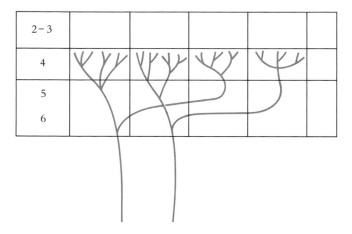

separated by 0.5-millimeter gaps, as shown in the illustration of synapse endings on this page. Because geniculate cells are monocular, any individual axon obviously belongs either to the left eye or the right eye. Suppose the green axon in the illustration is a left-eye fiber; it turns out that every left-eye fiber entering the cortex in this region will have its terminal branches in these same 0.5-millimeter clumps. Between the clumps, the 0.5-millimeter gaps are occupied by right-eye terminals. This special distribution of geniculo-cortical fibers in layer 4C explains at once the strict monocularity of cells in that layer.

To select one fiber and stain it and only it required a new method, first invented in the late 1970s. It is based on the phenomenon of axon transport. Materials, either proteins or larger particles, are constantly being transported, in both directions, along the interior of axons, some at rates measured in centimeters per hour, others at rates of about a millimeter per day. To stain a single axon, we inject it through a micropipette with a substance that is known to be transported and that will stain the axon without distorting the cell. The favorite substance at present is an enzyme called horseradish peroxidase. It is transported in both directions, and it catalyzes a chemical reaction that forms the basis of an exceedingly sensitive stain. Because it is a catalyst, minute amounts of it can generate a lot of stain and because it is of plant origin, none of it is normally around to give unwanted background staining.

The microelectrode penetrations in the vertical axis, by showing the cortex subdivided into ocular-dominance columns extending from the surface to the white matter, confirmed anatomical evidence that a patch of cells in layer 4C is the main supplier of visual information to cell layers above and below it. The existence of some horizontal and diagonal connections extending a millimeter or so in all directions must result in some smudging of the left-eye versus

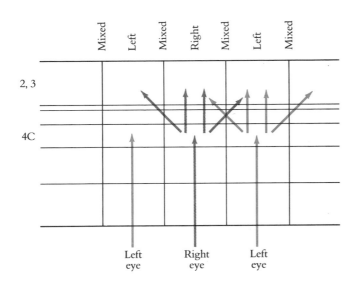

The overlap and blurring of ocular-dominance columns beyond layer 4 is due to horizontal or diagonal connections.

right-eye zones in the layers above and below 4C, as shown in the diagram on this page. We can expect that a cell sitting directly above the center of a layer-4 left-eye patch will therefore strongly favor that eye and perhaps be monopolized by it, whereas a cell closer to the border between two patches may be binocular and favor neither eye. Microelectrode penetrations that progress horizontally through one upper cortical layer, or through layer 5 or 6, recording cell after cell, do indeed find a progression of ocular dominance in which cells first favor one eye strongly, then less strongly, are then equally influenced, and then begin to favor the other eye progressively more strongly. This smooth alternation back and forth contrasts sharply with the sudden transitions we find if we advance the electrode through layer 4C.

Viewed from the side, the subdivisions in layer 4 appeared as patches. But

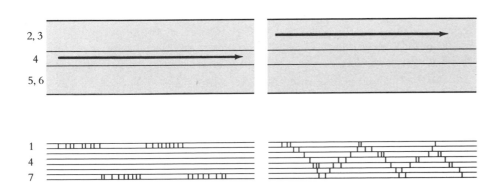

The ocular-dominance column borders in upper (2, 3) and lower (5, 6) layers are blurred, compared to the sharp boundaries in layer 4. The arrows illustrate electrode tracks made in layer 4 (upper left) and layer 2 or 3 (upper right). The lower diagrams plot ocular dominance of cells recorded along the tracks. In layer 4, we find abrupt alternation between group 1 (contralateral eye only) and group 7 (ipsilateral eye only). In other layers, we find binocular cells, and the eye dominance alternates by going through the intermediate degrees of eye preference. (1, 4, and 7 refer to ocular dominance.)

Here are three different ways that a surface can be partitioned off into two kinds of regions: the possible patterns are a checkerboard, stripes, and islands in an ocean. In this case, the surface is the cortex, and the regions are left-eye and right-eye.

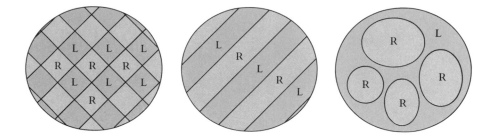

we wanted to know how the pattern would appear if we stood above the cortex and looked down. Suppose we have two regions, black and white, on a surface; topologically, we can partition them off in several different ways: in a checkerboard-like mosaic, in a series of black and white stripes, in black islands on a white ocean, or in any combination of these. The figures above show three possible patterns. To tackle the problem with microelectrodes alone amounts to using a one-dimensional technique to answer a three-dimensional question. That can be frustrating, like trying to cut the back lawn with a pair of nail scissors. One would prefer to switch to a completely different type of work, say farming, or the law. (In the early 1960s, when Torsten Weisel and I were more patient and determined, we actually did try to work out the geometry, with some success. And I actually did cut our back lawn once in those days, admittedly with kitchen scissors rather than nail scissors, because we could not afford a lawn mower. We were poorer than modern graduate students, but perhaps more patient.)

Luckily, neuroanatomical methods have been invented in breathtaking succession in the past decade, and by now the problem has been solved independently in about half a dozen ways. Here I will illustrate two.

The first method depends again on axon transport. A small amount of an organic chemical, perhaps an amino acid, is labeled with a radioactive element such as carbon-14 and injected into one eye of a monkey, say the left eye. The amino acid is taken up by the cells in the eye, including the retinal ganglion cells. The ganglion-cell axons transport the labeled molecule, presumably now incorporated into proteins, to their terminals in the lateral geniculate bodies. There the label accumulates in the left-eye layers. The process of transportation takes a few days. The tissue is then thinly sliced, coated with a photographic silver emulsion, and allowed to sit for some time in the dark. In the resulting autoradiograph, shown on the next page, we can see the three left-eye layers on each side, complementary in their order, revealed by black silver grains.

To see this geniculate pattern requires only modest amounts of radioactivity in the injection. If we inject a sufficiently large amount of the labeled amino

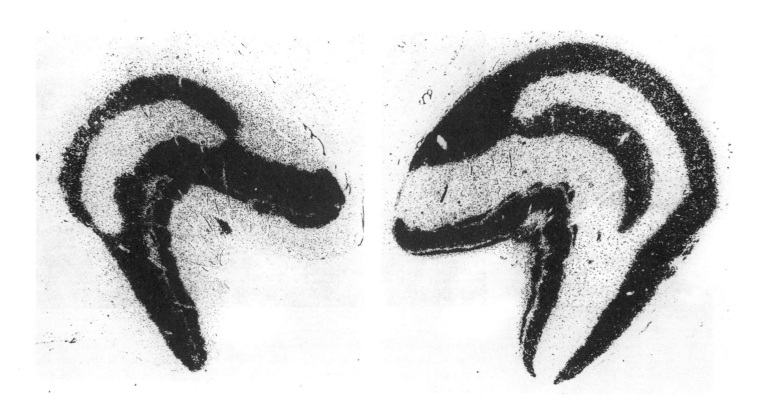

acid into the eye, the concentration in geniculate layers becomes so high that some radioactive material leaks out of the optic-nerve terminals and is taken up by the geniculate cells in the labeled layers and shipped along *their* axons to the striate cortex. The label thus accumulates in the layer-4C terminals in regular patches corresponding to the injected eye. When the autoradiograph is finally developed (after several months because the concentration of label finally reaching the cortex is very small), we can actually see the patches in layer 4C in a transverse section of the cortex, as shown in the photograph on the next page. If we slice the cortex parallel to its surface—either flattening it first or cutting and pasting serial sections—we can at last see the layout, as though we were viewing it from above. It is a beautiful set of parallel stripes, as shown on page III in a single section (top) and a reconstruction (bottom). In all these cortical autoradiographs, the label representing the left eye shows up bright, separated by dark, unlabeled regions representing the right eye. Because layer 4 feeds the layers above and below mainly by up-and-down connections, the regions of eye preference in three dimensions are a series of alternating left- and right-eye slabs, like slices of bread, as shown in the top diagram on page II2.

These sections through the left and right lateral geniculate bodies show autoradiographic label in the three left-eye layers on each side. The left eye had been injected with radioactive label (tritiated proline) a week earlier. The labeled layers are the dark ones.

In this autoradiograph through the striate cortex, the white segments are the labeled patches in layer 4 representing the injected left eye; these patches are separated by unlabeled (dark) right-eye regions.

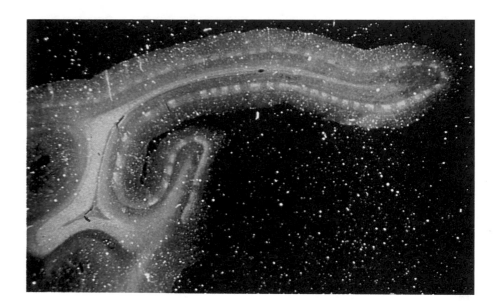

Using a different method, Simon LeVay succeeded in reconstructing the entire striate cortex in an occipital lobe; the part of this exposed on the surface is shown in the bottom illustration on page 112. The stripes of the pattern are most regular and striking some distance away from the foveal representation. For reasons unknown, the pattern is rather complex near the fovea, with very regular periodicity but many loops and swirls, hardly the regular wallpaper-like stripes seen farther out. The width of the stripes is everywhere constant at about 0.5 millimeter. The amount of cortex devoted to left and right eyes is nearly exactly equal in the cortex representing the fovea and out to about 20 degrees in all directions. LeVay and David Van Essen have found that owing to the declining contribution of the eye on the same side, the ipsilateral bands shrink to 0.25 millimeter out beyond 20 degrees from the fovea. Beyond 70 or 80 degrees, of course, only the contralateral eye is represented. This makes sense, because with your eyes facing the front, you can see with your right eye farther to the right than to the left.

A second method for demonstrating the columns reveals the slabs in their full thickness, not just the part in layer 4. This is the 2-deoxyglucose method, invented by Louis Sokoloff at the National Institutes of Health, Bethesda, in 1976. It too depends ultimately on the ability of radioactive substances to darken photographic film. The method is based on the fact that nerve cells, like most cells in the body, consume glucose as fuel, and the harder they are made to work, the more glucose they eat. Accordingly, we might imagine injecting radioactive glucose into an animal, stimulating one eye, say the

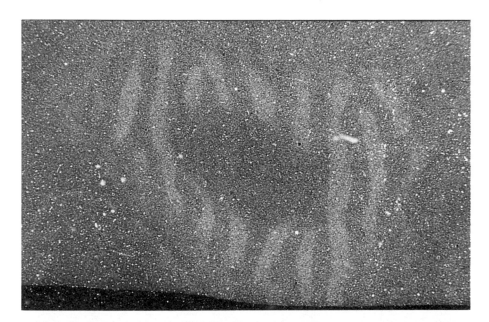

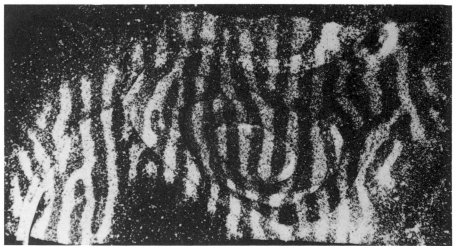

Top: A single section through the dome-shaped cortex is made parallel to the surface. It cuts through layer 4 in a ring. *Bottom:* A reconstruction of many such rings from a series of sections—the deeper the section, the bigger the ring—made by cutting out the rings and superimposing them. (Traces of the rings can be seen because it was difficult to get all the sections exposed and photographed equally, especially as I am strictly an amateur photographer.)

right, with patterns for some minutes—long enough for the glucose to be taken up by the active cells in the brain—and then removing the brain and slicing it, coating the slices with silver emulsion, and exposing and developing, as before. This idea didn't work because glucose is consumed by the cells and converted to energy and degradation products, which quickly leak back out into the blood stream. To sidestep the leakage, Sokoloff's ingenious trick

In three-dimensional view, the ocular-dominance columns are seen to be, not Greek pillars, but slabs perpendicular to the surface, like slices of bread.

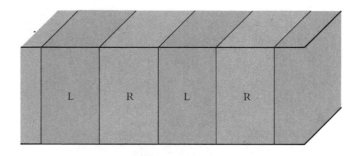

was to use the substance deoxyglucose, which is close enough chemically to glucose to fool the cells into taking it up: they even begin metabolizing it. The process of breakdown goes only one step along the usual chemical degradation path, coming to a halt after the deoxyglucose is converted to a substance (2-deoxyglucose-6-phosphate) that can be degraded no further. Luckily, this substance is fat insoluble and can't leak out of the cell; so it accumulates to levels at which it can be detected in autoradiographs. What we finally see on the film is a picture of the brain regions that became most active during the stimulation period and took up most of this fake food. Had the animal been moving its arm during that time, the motor arm area in the cortex would also have lit up. In the case of stimulating the right eye, what we see are the parts of the cortex most strongly activated by that stimulus, namely, the set of right

Seen here in LeVay's reconstruction are the ocular-dominance columns in the part of area 17 open to the surface, right hemisphere. Foveal representation is to the right. (Compare right side of photograph on page 95.)

5 mm

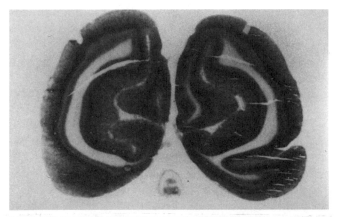

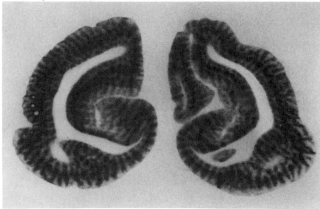

Two experiments using radioactive deoxyglucose. *Top:* A cross section of the two hemispheres through the occipital lobes in a control animal that had its visual field stimulated with both eyes open following the intravenous injection. *Bottom:* After injection, an animal viewed the stimulus with one eye open and the other closed. The ocular-dominance patterns are clearly visible in the cortex. This experiment was done by C. Kennedy, M. H. Des Rosiers, O. Sakurada, M. Shinohara, M. Reivich, J. W. Jehle, and L. Sokoloff.

ocular-dominance columns. You see the result in the photographs above.

In a very pretty extension of the same idea, Roger Tootell, in Russel De Valois's laboratory at Berkeley, had an animal look with one eye at a large pattern of concentric circles and rays, shown in the top image of the figure on the next page. The resulting pattern on the cortex contains the circles and rays, distorted just as expected by the variations in magnification (the distance on the cortex corresponding to 1 degree of visual field), a phenomenon related to the change in visual acuity between the fovea and periphery of the eye. Over and above that, each circle or ray is broken up by the fine ocular-dominance stripes. Stimulating both eyes would have resulted in continuous bands. Seldom can we illustrate so many separate facts so neatly, all in a single experiment.

Cats, several kinds of monkeys, chimpanzees, and man all possess ocular-dominance columns. The columns are absent in rodents and tree shrews; and although hints of their presence can be detected physiologically in the squirrel monkey, a new world monkey, present anatomical methods do not reveal the columns. At present we don't know what purpose this highly patterned segregation of eye influence serves, but one guess is that it has something to do with stereopsis (see Chapter 7).

Subdivisions of the cortex by specialization in cell function have been found in many regions besides the striate cortex. They were first seen in the somatosensory cortex by Vernon Mountcastle in the mid-1950s, in what was surely the most important set of observations on cortex since localization of function was first discovered. The somatosensory is to touch, pressure, and joint position what the striate cortex is to vision. Mountcastle showed that this cortex is similarly subdivided vertically into regions in which cells are sensitive to touch and regions in which cells respond to bending of joints or applying deep pressure to a limb. Like ocular-dominance columns, the regions are about half a

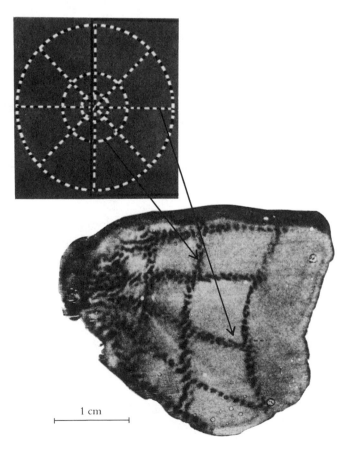

In this experiment by Roger Tootell, the target-shaped stimulus with radial lines was centered on an anesthetized macaque monkey's right visual field for 45 minutes after injection with radioactive 2-deoxyglucose. One eye was held closed. The lower picture shows the labeling in the striate cortex of the left hemisphere. This autoradiograph shows a section parallel to the surface; the cortex was flattened and frozen before sectioning. The roughly vertical lines of label represent the (semi)circular stimulus lines; the horizontal lines of label represent the radial lines in the right visual field. The hatching within each line of label is caused by only one eye having been stimulated and represents ocular-dominance columns.

1 cm

millimeter across, but whether they form stripes, a checkerboard, or an ocean-and-islands pattern is still not clear. The term *column* was coined by Mountcastle, so one can probably assume that he had a pillarlike structure in mind. We now know that the word *slab* would be more suitable for the visual cortex. Terminology is hard to change, however, and it seems best to stick to the well-known term, despite its shortcomings. Today we speak of *columnar subdivisions* when some cell attribute remains constant from surface to white matter and varies in records taken parallel to the surface. For reasons that will become clear in the next chapter, we usually restrict the concept to exclude the topographic representation, that is, position of receptive fields on the retina or position on the body.

ORIENTATION COLUMNS

In the earliest recordings from the striate cortex, it was noticed that whenever two cells were recorded together, they agreed not only in their eye preference, but also in their preferred orientation. You might reasonably ask at this point whether next-door neighboring cells agree in all their properties: the answer is clearly no. As I have mentioned, receptive-field positions are usually not quite the same, although they usually overlap; directional preferences are often opposite, or one cell may show a marked directional preference and the other show none. In layers 2 and 3, where end-stopping is found, one cell may show no stopping when its neighbor is completely stopped. In contrast, it is very rare for two cells recorded together to have opposite eye preference or any obvious difference in orientation.

Orientation, like eye preference, remains constant in vertical penetrations through the full cortical thickness. In layer $4C\beta$, as described earlier, cells show no orientation preference at all, but as soon as we reach layer 5, the cells show strong orientation preference and the preferred orientation is the same as it was above layer 4C. If we pull out the electrode and reinsert it somewhere else, the whole sequence of events is seen again, but a different orientation very likely will prevail. The cortex is thus subdivided into slender regions of constant orientation, extending from surface to white matter but interrupted by layer 4, where cells have no orientation preference.

If, on the other hand, the electrode is pushed through the cortex in a direction parallel to the surface, an amazingly regular sequence of changes in orientation occurs: every time the electrode advances 0.05 millimeter (50 micrometers), on the average the preferred orientation shifts about 10 degrees clockwise or counterclockwise. Consequently a traverse of 1 millimeter typically records a total shift of 180 degrees. Fifty micrometers and 10 degrees are close to the

A very oblique penetration through area 17 in a macaque monkey reveals the regular shift in orientation preference of 23 neighboring cells.

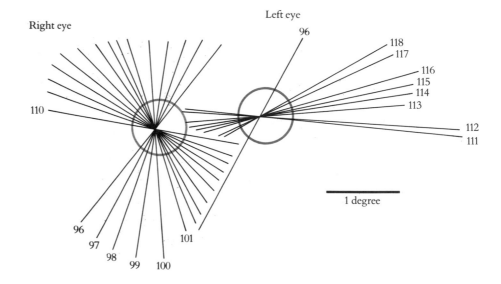

present limits of the precision of measurements, so that it is impossible to say whether orientation varies in any sense continuously with electrode position, or shifts in discrete steps.

In the two figures on this page and the next, a typical experiment is illustrated for part of a close-to-horizontal penetration through area 17, in which 23 cells were recorded. The eyes were not perfectly aligned on the screen (because of the anesthetic and a muscle-relaxing agent), so that the projections of the foveas of the two eyes were separated by about 2 degrees. The color circles in the figure above represent roughly the sizes of the receptive fields, about a degree in diameter, positioned 4 degrees below and to the left of the foveal projections—the records were from the right hemisphere. The first cell, 96, was binocular, but the next 14 were dominated strongly by the right eye. From then on, for cells 111 to 118, the left eye took over. You can see how regularly the orientations were shifting during this sequence, in this case always counterclockwise. When the shift in orientation is plotted against track distance (in the graph on the next page), the points form an almost perfect straight line. The change from one eye to the other was not accompanied by any obvious change either in the tendency to shift counterclockwise or in the slope of the line. We interpret this to mean that the two systems of groupings, by eye dominance and by orientation, are not closely related. It is as though the cortex were diced up in two completely different ways.

In such penetrations, the direction of orientation shifts may be clockwise or counterclockwise, and most penetrations, if long enough, sooner or later show shifts in the direction of rotation; these occur at unpredictable intervals of a

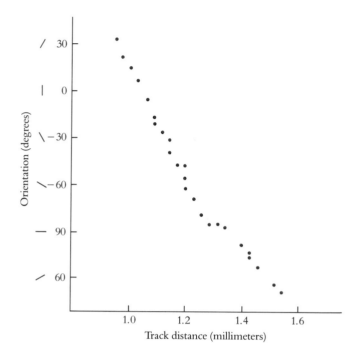

The results of the experiment shown on the facing page are plotted in degrees, against the distance the electrode had traveled. (Because the electrode was so slanted that it was almost parallel to the cortical surface, the track distance is almost the same as the distance along the surface.) In this experiment 180 degrees, a full rotation, corresponded to about 0.7 millimeter.

few millimeters. The graph on the next page shows an example of a sequence with several such reversals.

We see in some experiments a final peculiarity called a *fracture*. Just as we are becoming mesmerized by the relentless regularity, observing shift after shift in the same direction, we see on rare occasions a sudden break in the sequence, with a shift of 45 to 90 degrees. The sequence then resumes with the same regularity, but often with a reversal from clockwise to counterclockwise. The graph on page 119 shows such a fracture, followed a few tenths of a millimeter later by another one.

The problem of learning what these groupings, or regions of constant orientation, look like if viewed from above the cortex has proved much more difficult than viewing ocular-dominance columns from the same perspective. Until very recently we have had no direct way of seeing the orientation groupings and have had to try to deduce the form from microelectrode penetrations such as those I have shown here. The reversals and fractures both suggest that the geometry is not simple. On the other hand, the linear regularity that we see, often over millimeter after millimeter of cortex, must imply a regularity at least within small regions of cortex; the reversals and fractures would then suggest that the regularity is broken up every few millimeters.

In still another experiment where we graph orientation against track distance, three reversals separated long, straight progressions.

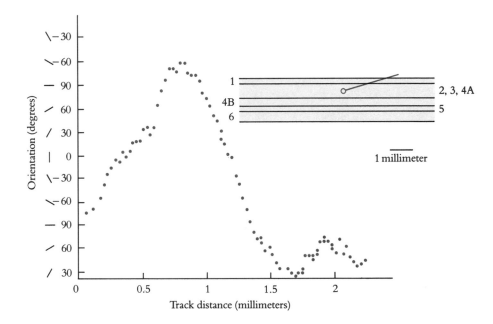

Within these regions of regularity, we can predict the geometry to some extent. Suppose that the region is such that wherever we explore it with an electrode parallel to the surface, we see regularity—no reversals and no fractures—that is, everywhere we obtain graphs like the one on page 117. If we had enough of these graphs, we could ultimately construct a three-dimensional graph, as in the illustration shown on the facing page, with orientation represented on a vertical axis (z) plotted against cortical distance on horizontal axes (x and y). Orientations would then be represented on a surface such as the tilted plane in this illustration, in cases where the graphs were straight lines, and otherwise on some kind of curved surface. In this three-dimensional graph horizontal planes (the x-y plane or planes parallel to it) would intersect this surface in lines, contour lines of constant orientation (iso-orientation lines) analogous to lines of constant height in a contour map in geography. Undulations—hills, valleys, ridges—in the 3-D graph would give reversals in some orientation-versus-distance plots; sudden breaks in the form of cliffs would lead to the fractures. The main message from this argument is that regions of regularity imply the possibility of plotting a contour map, which means that regions of constant orientation, seen looking down on the cortex from above, must be stripes. Because orientations plotted in vertical penetrations through the cortex are constant, the regions in three dimensions must be slabs. And because the iso-orientation lines may curve, the slabs need not be flat like slices of bread. Much of this has been demonstrated directly in experiments making

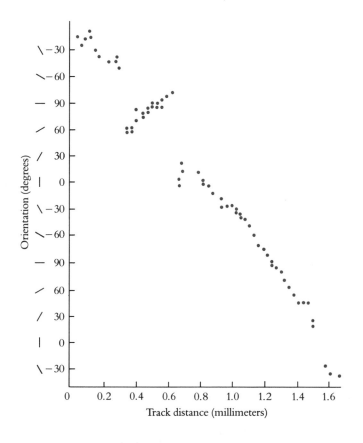

This penetration showed two fractures, or sudden shifts in orientation, following and followed by regular sequences of shifts.

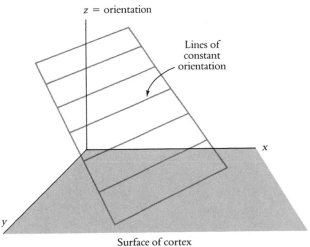

The surface of the cortex is plotted on the x-y plane in this three dimensional map; the vertical (z) axis represents orientation. If for all directions of electrode tracks straight line orientation-versus-distance plots are produced, the surface generated will be a plane, and intersections of the surface (whether planar or not) with the x-y plane, and planes parallel to it, will give contour lines. (This sounds more complicated than it is! The same reasoning applies if the x-y plane is the surface of Tierra del Fuego and the z axis represents altitude or average rainfall in January or temperature.)

two or three parallel penetrations less than a millimeter apart, and the three-dimensional form has been reconstructed at least over those tiny volumes.

If our reasoning is right, occasional penetrations should occur in the same direction as contour lines, and orientation should be constant. This does happen, but not very often. That, too, is what we would predict, because trigonometry tells us that a small departure from a contour line, in a penetration's direction, gives a rather large change in slope, so that few graphs of orientation versus distance should be very close to horizontal.

The number of degrees of orientation represented in a square millimeter of cortex should be given by the steepest slopes that we find. This is about 400 degrees per millimeter, which means a full complement of 180 degrees of orientation in about 0.5 millimeter. This is a number to have in mind when we return to contemplate the topography of the cortex and its striking uniformity. Here, I cannot resist pointing out that the thickness of a pair of ocular-dominance columns is 0.4 plus 0.4 millimeter, or roughly 1 millimeter, double, but about the same order of magnitude, as the set of orientation slabs.

Deoxyglucose mapping was soon seized on as a direct way of determining orientation-column geometry. We simply stimulated with parallel stripes, keeping orientation constant, say vertical, for the entire period of stimulation. The pattern we obtained, as shown in the top autoradiograph on the facing page, was far more complex than that of ocular-dominance columns. Nevertheless the periodicity was clear, with 1 millimeter or less from one dense region to the next, as would be expected from the physiology—the distance an electrode has to move to go from a given orientation, such as vertical, through all intermediates and back to vertical. Some places showed stripelike regularity extending for several square millimeters. We had wondered whether the orientation slabs and the ocular-dominance stripes might in any way be related in their geometry—for example, be parallel or intersect at 90 degrees. In the same experiment, we were able to reveal the ocular-dominance columns by injecting the eye with a radioactive amino acid and to look at the same block of tissue by the two methods, as shown in the second autoradiograph on the facing page. We could see no obvious correlation. Given the complex pattern of the orientation domains, compared with the relatively much simpler pattern of the ocular-dominance columns, it was hard to see how the two patterns *could* be closely related.

For some types of questions the deoxyglucose method has a serious limitation. It is hard always to be sure that the pattern we obtain is really related to whatever stimulus variable we have used. For example, using black and white vertical stripes as a stimulus, how can we be sure the pattern is caused by verticality—that the dark areas contain cells responding to vertical, the light areas, cells responding to nonvertical? The features of the stimulus responsible for the pattern could be the use of black-white, as opposed to color, or the use of coarse stripes, as opposed to fine ones, or the placing of the screen at some

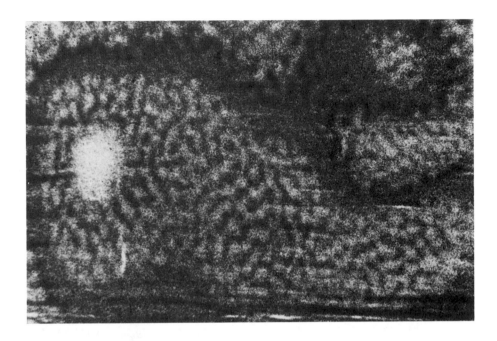

After the injection of deoxyglucose, the visual fields of the anesthetized monkey were stimulated with slowly moving vertical black and white stripes. The resulting autoradiograph shows dense periodic labeling, for example in layers 5 and 6 (large central elongated area). The dark gray narrow ring outside this, layer 4Cβ, is uniformly labeled, as expected, because the cells are not orientation selective.

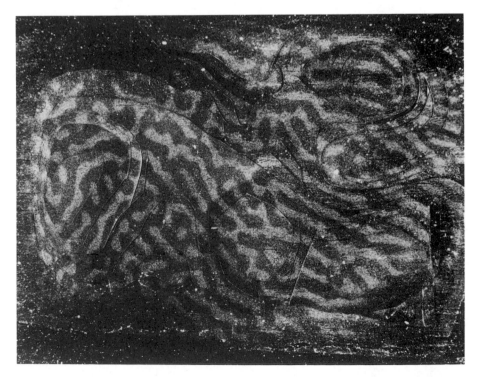

In the same animal as above, one eye had been injected a week earlier with radioactive amino acid (proline), and after washing the section in water to dissolve the 2-deoxyglucose, an autoradiograph was prepared from the same region as in the upper autoradiograph. Label shows ocular-dominance columns. These have no obvious relationship to the orientation columns.

particular distance rather than another. One indirect confirmation that orientation is involved in the deoxyglucose work is the absence of any patchiness or periodicities in layer 4C, where cells lack orientation preference. Another comes from a study in which Michael Stryker, at the University of California at San Fransisco, made long microelectrode penetrations parallel to the surface in cat striate cortex, planted lesions every time some particular orientation was encountered, and finally stimulated with stripes of one orientation after injecting radioactive deoxyglucose. These experiments showed a clear correlation between the pattern and stimulus orientation.

The most dramatic demonstration of orientation columns comes from the use of voltage-sensitive dyes, developed over many years by Larry Cohen at Yale and applied to the cerebral cortex by Gary Blasdel at the University of Pittsburgh. In this technique, a voltage-sensitive dye that stains cell membranes is poured onto the cortex of an anesthetized animal and is taken up by the nerve cells. When an animal is stimulated, any responding cells show slight changes in color, and if enough cells are affected in a region close enough to the surface, we can record these changes with modern TV imaging techniques and computer-aided noise filtration. Blasdel stimulated with stripes in some particular orientation, made a photograph of the pattern of activity in a region of cortical surface a few centimeters in area, and repeated the procedure for

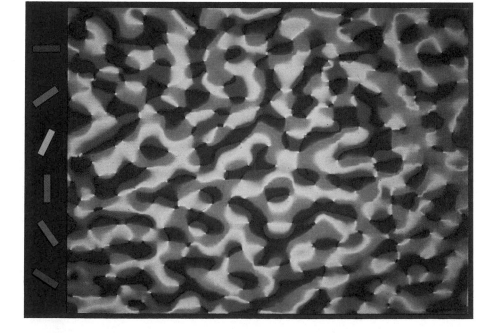

In this experiment Gary Blasdel applied a voltage-sensitive dye to a monkey's striate cortex and stimulated the visual fields with stripes of one orientation after the next, while imaging the cortex with TV techniques. Using computers, the results are displayed by assigning a color to each set of regions lit up by each orientation. For any small region of cortex the orientation slabs are parallel stripes, so that a complete set of orientations appears as a tiny rainbow.

many orientations. He then assigned a color to each orientation—red for vertical, orange for one o'clock, and so on—and superimposed the pictures. Because an iso-orientation line should be progressively displaced sideways as orientation changes, the result in any one small region should be a rainbowlike pattern. This is exactly what Blasdell found. It is too early, and the number of examples are still too few, to allow an interpretation of the patterns in terms of fractures and reversals, but the method is promising.

MAPS OF THE CORTEX

Now that we know something about the mapping of orientation and ocular-dominance parameters onto the cortex, we can begin to consider the relation between these maps and the projections of the visual fields. It used to be said that the retina mapped to the cortex in point-to-point fashion, but given what we know about the receptive fields of cortical cells, it is clear that this cannot be true in any strict sense: each cell receives input from thousands of rods and cones, and its receptive field is far from being a point. The map from retina to cortex is far more intricate than any simple point-to-point map. I have tried in the figure on the next page to map the distribution of regions on the cortex that are activated by a simple stimulus (not to be confused with the receptive field of a single cell). The stimulus is a short line tilted at 60 degrees to the vertical, presented to the left eye only. We suppose that this part of the visual field projects to the area of cortex indicated by the rounded-corner rectangle. Within that area, only left-eye slabs will be activated, and of these, only 60-degree slabs; these are filled in in black in the illustration. So a line in the visual field produces a bizarre distribution of cortical activity in the form, roughly, of an array of bars.

Now you can begin to see how silly it is to imagine a little green man sitting up in our head, contemplating such a pattern. The pattern that the cortex happens to display is about as relevant as the pattern of activity of a video camera's insides, wires and all, in response to an outside scene. The pattern of activity on the cortex is anything but a reproduction of the outside scene. If it were, that would mean only that nothing interesting had happened between eye and cortex, in which case we would indeed need a little green man.

We can hardly imagine that nature would have gone to the trouble of grouping cells so beautifully in these two independently coexisting sets of columns if it were not of some advantage to the animal. Until we work out the exact wiring responsible for the transformations that occur in the cortex, we are not likely to understand the groupings completely. At this point we can only make logical guesses. If we suppose the circuits proposed in Chapter 4 are at all close

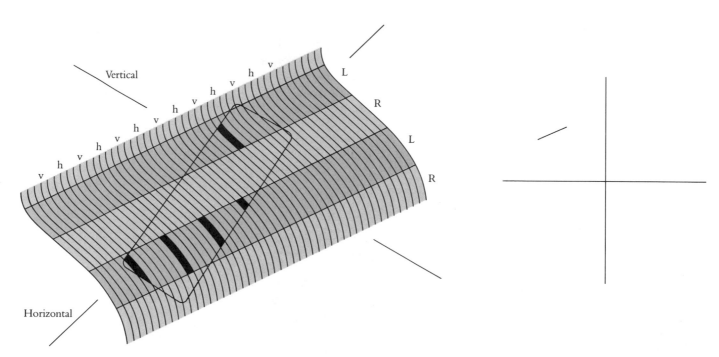

A tilted line segment shining in the visual field of the left eye (shown to the right) may cause this hypothetical pattern of activation of a small area of striate cortex (shown to the left). The activation is confined to a small cortical area, which is long and narrow to reflect the shape of the line; within this area, it is confined to left ocular-dominance columns and to orientation columns representing a two o'clock–eight o'clock tilt. Cortical representation is not simple! When we consider that the orientation domains are not neat parallel lines, suggested here for simplicity, but far more complex, as shown in the upper, deoxyglucose figure on page 121 and Blasdel's figure on page 122, the representation becomes even more intricate.

to reality, then what is required to build complex cells from simple ones, or to accomplish end-stopping or directional selectivity, is in each case a convergence of many cells onto a single cell, with all the interconnected cells having the same receptive-field orientation and roughly the same positions. So far, we have no compelling reasons to expect that a cell with some particular receptive-field orientation should receive inputs from cells with different orientations. (I am exaggerating a bit: suggestions have been made that cells of different orientation affiliations might be joined by inhibitory connections: the evidence for such connections is indirect and as yet, to my mind, not very strong, but it is not easily dismissed.) If this is so, why not group together the cells that are to be interconnected? The alternative is hardly attractive: imagine the problem of having to wire together the appropriate cells if they were scattered through the cortex without regard to common properties. By far the densest interconnections should be between cells having common orientations; if cells were distributed at random, without regard to orientation, the tangle of axons necessary to interconnect the appropriate cells would be massive. As it is, they are, in fact, grouped together. The same argument applies to ocular-dominance domains.

If the idea is to pack cells with like properties together, why have sequences of small orientation steps? And why the cycles? Why go through all possible orientations and then come back to the first, and cycle around again, instead of

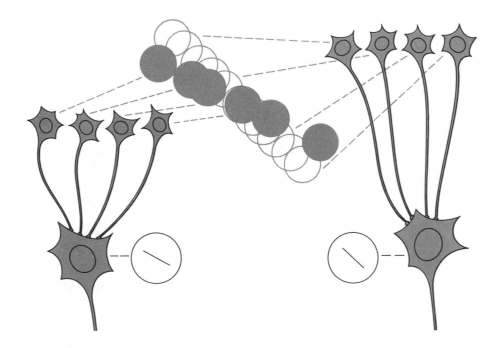

The group of center-surround layer 4 cells that is needed to build a simple cell that responds to an oblique four o'clock–ten o'clock slit is likely to have cells in common with the group needed to build a 4:30–10:30 cell: a few inputs must be discarded and a few added.

packing together *all* cells with 30-degree orientation, all cells with 42-degree orientation, and indeed all left-eye cells and all right-eye cells? Given that we know how the cortex *is* constructed, we can suggest many answers. Here is one suggestion: perhaps cells of unlike orientation do indeed inhibit one another. We do not want a cell to respond to orientations other than its own, and we can easily imagine that inhibitory connections result in a sharpening of orientation tuning. The existing system is then just what is wanted: cells are physically closest to cells of like orientation but are not too far away from cells of almost the same orientation; the result is that the inhibitory connections do not have to be very long. A second suggestion: if we consider the connections necessary to build a simple cell with some particular opitimal orientation out of a group of center-surround layer-4 cells, more or less the same inputs will be required to build a nearby simple cell with a different, but not a very different, orientation. The correct result will be obtained if we add a few inputs and drop a few, as suggested in the illustration on this page. Something like that might well justify the proximity of cells with similar orientations.

The topic to be considered in the next chapter, the relationship between orientation, ocular dominance, and the projection of visual fields onto the cortex, may help us understand why so many columns should be desirable. When we add topography into the equation, the intricacy of the system increases in a fascinating way.

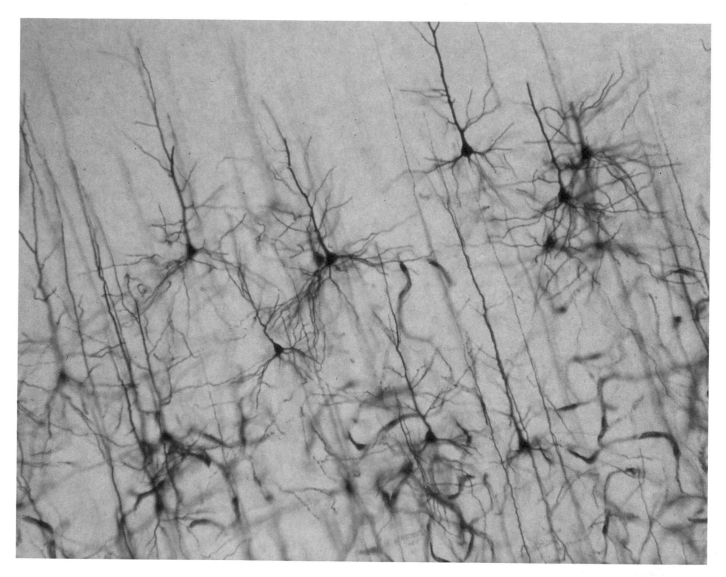

A single module of the type discussed in this chapter occupies roughly the area shown in this photograph of a Golgi-stained section through visual cortex. The Golgi method stains only a tiny fraction of the nerve cells in any region, but the cells that it does reveal are stained fully or almost so; thus one can see the cell body, dendrites, and axon.

6

MAGNIFICATION AND MODULES

In the last chapter I emphasized the uniformity of the anatomy of the cortex, as it appears to the naked eye and even, with most ordinary staining methods, under the microscope. Now, on closer inspection, we have found anatomical uniformity prevailing in the topography of the ocular-dominance columns: the repeat distance, from left eye to right eye, stays remarkably constant as we go from the fovea to the far periphery of the binocular region. With the help of the deoxyglucose method and optical mapping techniques, we have found uniformity in the topography of the orientation columns as well.

This uniformity came at first as a surprise, because functionally the visual cortex is decidedly nonuniform, in two important respects. First, as described in Chapter 3, the receptive fields of retinal ganglion cells in or near the fovea are much smaller than those of cells many degrees out from the fovea. In the cortex, the receptive field of a typical complex upper-layer cell in the foveal representation is about one-quarter to one-half a degree in length and width. If we go out to 80 or 90 degrees, the comparable dimensions are more like 2 to 4 degrees—a ratio, in area, of about 10 to 30.

The second kind of nonuniformity concerns *magnification*, defined in 1961 by P. M. Daniel and David Whitteridge as the distance in the cortex corresponding to a distance of 1 degree in the visual field. As we go out from the fovea, a given amount of visual field corresponds to a progressively smaller and smaller area of cortex: the magnification decreases. If, near the fovea, we move 1 degree in the visual field, we travel about 6 millimeters on the cortex; 90 degrees out from the fovea, 1 degree in the visual field corresponds to about 0.15 millimeter along the cortex. Thus magnification in the fovea is roughly thirty-six times larger than in the periphery.

Both these nonuniformities make sense—and for the same reason—namely, that our vision gets progressively cruder with distance from the fovea. Just try looking at a letter at the extreme left of this page and guessing at any letter or word at the extreme right. Or look at the word *progressively*: if you fix your gaze on the *p* at the beginning, you may just barely be able to see the *y* at the end, and you will certainly have trouble with the *e* or the *l* before the *y*. Achieving high resolution in the foveal part of our visual system requires many cortical cells per unit area of visual field, with each cell taking care of a very small domain of visual field.

THE SCATTER AND DRIFT OF RECEPTIVE FIELDS

How, then, can the cortex get away with being so uniform anatomically? To understand this we need to take a more detailed look at what happens to receptive-field positions as an electrode moves through the cortex. If the electrode is inserted into the striate cortex exactly perpendicular to the surface, the receptive fields of cells encountered as the tip moves forward are all located in almost the same place, but not exactly: from cell to cell we find variations in position, which seem to be random and are small enough that some overlap occurs between almost every field and the next one, as shown in the illustration on this page. The sizes of the fields remain fairly constant in any given layer but differ markedly from one layer to another, from very small, in layer 4C, to large, in layers 5 and 6. Within any one layer, the area of visual field occupied by ten or twenty successively recorded receptive fields is, because of this random scatter, about two to four times the area occupied by any single field. We call the area occupied by a large number of superimposed fields in some layer and under some point on the cortex the *aggregate receptive field* of that point in that layer. In any given layer, the aggregate field varies, for example in layer 3, from about 30 minutes of arc in the foveal region to about 7 or 8 degrees in the far periphery.

Now suppose we insert the electrode so that it moves horizontally along any one layer, say layer 3. Again, as cell after cell is recorded, we see in successive receptive fields a chaotic variation in position, but superimposed on this variation we now detect a steady drift in position. The direction of this drift in the visual field is, of course, predictable from the systematic map of visual fields onto cortex. What interests us here is the amount of drift we see after 1 millimeter of horizontal movement along the cortex. From what I have said about variation in magnification, it will be clear that the distance traversed in the visual field will depend on where in the cortex we have been recording—whether we are studying a region of cortex that represents the foveal region, the far periphery of the visual field, or somewhere between. The rate of movement through the visual field will be far from constant. But the movement turns out to be very constant relative to the size of the receptive fields them-

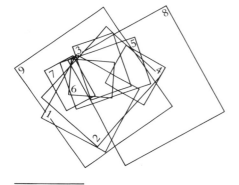

1 degree

These nine receptive fields were mapped in a cat striate cortex in a single microelectrode penetration made perpendicular to the surface. As the electrode descends, we see random scatter in receptive-field position and some variation in size but see no overall tendency for the positions to change.

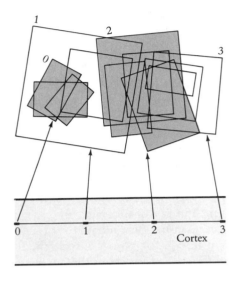

1 degree

In the course of a long penetration parallel to the cortical surface in a cat, receptive fields drifted through the visual field. The electrode traveled over 3 millimeters and recorded over sixty cells, far too many to be shown in a figure like this. I show instead only the positions of four or five receptive fields mapped in the first tenth of each millimeter, ignoring the other nine-tenths. For the parts of the penetration drawn with a thick pen in the lower half of the diagram (numbered 0, 1, 2, and 3), the receptive fields of cells encountered are mapped in the upper part. Each group is detectably displaced to the right in the visual field relative to the previous group. The fields in group 2 do not overlap with those in group 0, and group-3 fields do not overlap with group-1 fields; in each case the cortical separation is 2 millimeters.

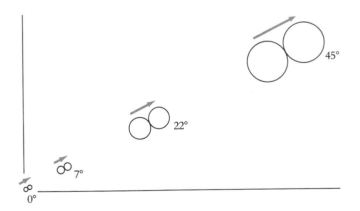

In a macaque monkey, the upper-layer receptive fields grow larger as eccentricity increases from the fovea (0 degrees). Also growing by an equal amount is the distance the receptive fields move in the visual field when an electrode moves 2 millimeters along the cortex parallel to the surface.

selves. One millimeter on the cortex everywhere produces a movement through the visual field that is equal to about half the territory occupied by the aggregate receptive field—the smear of fields that would be found under a single point in the region. Thus about 2 millimeters of movement is required to get entirely out of one part of the visual field and into the next, as shown in the illustration at the top of this page. This turns out to be the case wherever in area 17 we record. In the fovea, the receptive fields are tiny, and so is the movement in the visual field produced by a 2-millimeter movement along the cortex: in the periphery, both the receptive fields and the movements are much larger, as illustrated in the lower figure on this page.

UNITS OF FUNCTION
IN THE CORTEX

We must conclude that any piece of primary visual cortex about 2 millimeters by 2 millimeters in surface area must have the machinery to deal completely with some particular area of visual field—an area of visual field that is small in or near the fovea and large in the periphery. A piece of cortex receiving input from perhaps a few tens of thousands of fibers from the geniculate first operates on the information and then supplies an output carried by fibers sensitive to orientation, movement, and so on, combining the information from the two eyes: each such piece does roughly the same set of operations on about the same number of incoming fibers. It takes in information, highly detailed over a small visual-field terrain for fovea but coarser and covering a larger visual-field terrain for points outside the fovea, and it emits an output—without knowing or caring about the degree of detail or the size of the visual field it subserves. The machinery is everywhere much the same. That explains the uniformity observed in the gross and microscopic anatomy.

The fact that covering a 2-millimeter span of cortex is just enough to move you into a completely new area of retina means that whatever local operations are to be done by the cortex must all be done within this 2 millimeter by 2 millimeter chunk. A smaller piece of cortex is evidently not adequate to deal with a correspondingly smaller retinal terrain, since the rest of the 2-millimeter piece is also contributing to the analysis of that region. This much is obvious simply from a consideration of receptive-field positions and sizes, but the point can be amplified by asking in more detail what is meant by *analysis* and *operation*. We can start by considering line orientation. For any region in the visual field, however small, all orientations must be taken care of. If in analyzing a piece of retina, a 2-millimeter piece of cortex fails to take care of the orientation +45 degrees, no other part of the cortex can make up the deficit, because other parts are dealing with other parts of the visual field. By great good luck, however, the widths of the orientation stripes in the cortex, 0.05 millimeter, are just small enough that with 180 degrees to look after in 10-degree steps, all orientations can be covered comfortably, more than twice over, in 2 millimeters. The same holds for eye dominance: each eye requires 0.5 millimeter, so that 2 millimeters is more than enough. In a 2-millimeter block, the cortex seems to possess, as indeed it must, a complete set of machinery.

Let me hasten to add that the 2-millimeter distance is a property not so much of area 17 as of layer 3 in area 17. In layers 5 and 6, the fields and the scatter are twice the size, so that a block roughly 4 millimeters by 4 millimeters would presumably be needed to do everything layers 5 and 6 do, such as constructing big complex fields with rather special properties. At the other extreme, in

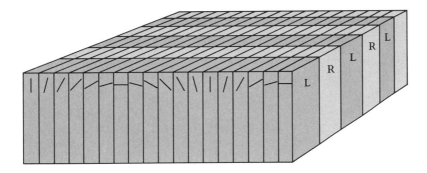

We call this our "ice cube model" of the cortex. It illustrates how the cortex is divided, at one and the same time, into two kinds of slabs, one set for ocular dominance (left and right) and one set for orientation. The model should not be taken literally: Neither set is as regular as this, and the orientation slabs especially are far from parallel or straight. Moreover, they do not seem to intersect in any particular angle—certainly they are not orthogonal, as shown here.

layer 4C, fields and scatter are far smaller, and the corresponding distance in the cortex is more like 0.1 to 0.2 millimeter. But the general argument remains the same, unaffected by the fact that several local sets of operations are made on any given region of visual field in several different layers—that is, despite the fact that the cortex is several machines in one.

All this may help us to understand why the columns are not far more coarse. Enough has to be packed into a 2 millimeter by 2 millimeter block to include all the values of the variables it deals with, orientation and eye preference being the ones we have talked about so far. What the cortex does is map not just two but many variables on its two-dimensional surface. It does this by selecting as the basic parameters the two variables that specify the visual field coordinates (distance out and up or down from the fovea), and on this map it engrafts other variables, such as orientation and eye preference, by finer subdivisions.

We call the 2 millimeter by 2 millimeter piece of cortex a *module*. To me, the word seems not totally suitable, partly because it is too concrete: it calls up an image of a rectangular tin box containing electronic parts that can be plugged into a rack beside a hundred other such boxes. To some extent that is indeed what we want the word to convey, but in a rather loose sense. First, our units clearly can start and end anywhere we like, in the orientation domain. They can go from vertical to vertical or −85 to +95 degrees, as long as we include all orientations at least once. The same applies to eye preference: we can start at a left-eye, right-eye border or at the middle of a column, as long as we include two columns, one for each eye. Second, as mentioned earlier, the size of the module we are talking about will depend on the layer we are considering. Nevertheless, the term does convey the impression of some 500 to 1000 small machines, any of which can be substituted for any other, provided we are ready to wire up 10,000 or so incoming wires and perhaps 50,000 outgoing ones!

Let me quickly add that no one would suppose that the cortex is completely uniform from fovea to far periphery. Vision varies with visual-field position in several ways other than acuity. Our color abilities fall off with distance, although perhaps not very steeply if we compensate for magnification by making the object we are viewing bigger with increasing distance from the fovea. Movement is probably better detected in the periphery, as are very dim lights. Functions related to binocular vision must obviously fall off because beyond 20 degrees and up to 80 degrees, ipsilateral-eye columns get progressively narrower and contralateral ones get broader; beyond 80 degrees the ipsilateral ones disappear entirely and the cortex becomes monocular. There must be differences in circuits to reflect these and doubtless other differences in our capabilities. So modules are probably not all exactly alike.

DEFORMATION OF THE CORTEX

We can get a deeper understanding of the geometry of the cortex by comparing it with the retina. The eye is a sphere, and that is consequently the shape of the retina, for purely optical reasons. A camera film can be flat because the angle taken in by the system is, for an average lens, about 30 degrees. A fish-eye camera lens encompasses a wider angle, but it distorts at the periphery. Of course, bowl-shaped photographs would be awkward—flat ones are enough of a pain to store. For the eye, a spherical shape is ideal, since a sphere is compact and can rotate in a socket, something that a cube does with difficulty! With a spherical eye, retinal magnification is constant: the number of degrees of visual field per millimeter of retina is the same throughout the retina—3.5 degrees per millimeter in human eyes. I have already mentioned that ganglion-cell receptive-field centers are small in and near the fovea and grow in size as distance from fovea increases, and accordingly we should not be surprised to learn that many more ganglion cells are needed in a millimeter of retina near the fovea than are needed far out. Indeed, near the fovea, ganglion cells are piled many cells high, whereas the cells farther out are spread too thin to make even one continuous layer, as the photographs on the facing page show. Because the retina has to be spherical, its layers cannot be uniform. Perhaps that is part of the reason for the retina's not doing more information processing than it does. The layers near the fovea would have to be much too thick.

The cortex has more options. Unlike the retina, it does not have to be spherical; it is allowed simply to expand in its foveal part, relative to the periphery. It presumably expands enough so that the thickness—and incidentally the column widths and everything else—remains the same throughout.

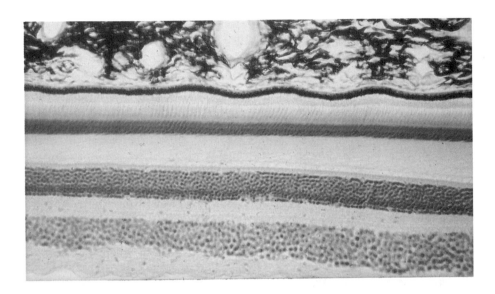

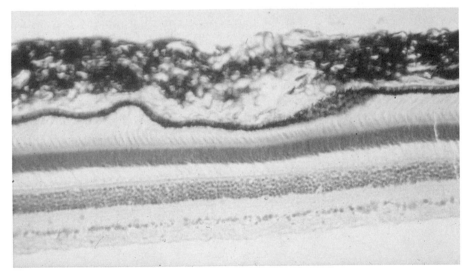

In contrast to those of the cortex, the layers of the retina are far from constant in thickness. In both monkey and human the ganglion-cell layer near the fovea (bottom layer, top photograph) is many cell bodies thick, perhaps eight or ten, whereas far in the periphery, say 70 to 80 degrees out, (bottom photograph) there are too few ganglion cells to make one layer. This should be no surprise since foveal ganglion-cell field centers are tiny; they are larger in the periphery (just as in the cortex). Thus in the fovea, compared with the periphery, it takes more cells to look after a unit area of retina.

How does this affect the overall shape of the striate cortex? Although I have repeatedly called the cortex a plate, I have not necessarily meant to imply that it is a plane. If there were no distortion at all in shape, the striate cortex would be a sphere, just as the eyeball is and just as any map of the earth, if undistorted, must be. (Strictly, of course, the striate cortex on one side maps about half of the back halves of the two eyes, or about a quarter-sphere.) In stretching, so as to keep thickness constant and yet manage many more messages from the crowded layers of ganglion cells at the fovea, the cortex becomes distorted relative to the spherical surface that it otherwise would approximate. If we unfold and smooth out the creases in the cortex, we discover that it is indeed neither spherical nor flat; it has the shape of a very distorted quarter-sphere, rather like a pear or an egg. This result was predicted in 1962 by Daniel and Whitteridge, who determined experimentally the magnification in area 17 as a function of distance from the foveal representation, as mentioned on page 127, and used the result to calculate the three-dimensional shape. They then made a rubber model of the cortex from serial histological sections and literally unfolded it, thus verifying the pear shape they had predicted. We can see the shape in the illustration on this page. Till then no one had reasoned out the question so as to predict that the cortex would unfold into any reasonable shape, nor, to my knowledge, had anyone realized that for any area of cortex, *some* shape or other must exist whose configuration should follow logically from its function. Presumably the folds, which must be smoothed out (without stretching or tearing) to get at the essential shape, exist because this large, distorted quarter-sphere must be crumpled to fit the compact box of the skull. The foldings may not be entirely arbitrary: some of the details are probably determined so as to minimize the lengths of cortico-cortical connections.

The unfolded striate cortex has a shape something like a pear. It would be a quarter-sphere if the visual fields were equally represented everywhere, but instead it is greatly distorted by the disproportionate representation of parts near the center of gaze (retinal fovea). The far periphery, almost 90 degrees out, is so underrepresented that the half circle corresponding to 90 degrees, at the extreme right in the figure, is very small.

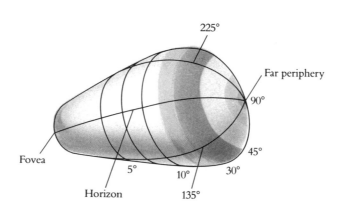

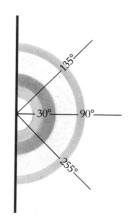

In the somatosensory cortex the problems of topography can become extreme to the point of absurdity. The cortex corresponding to the skin covering the hand, for example, should have basically a glove shape, with distortions over and above that to allow for the much greater sensory capacities of the finger tips, as compared with the palm or back of the hand. Such a distortion is analogous to the distortion of the foveal projections relative to the periphery, to allow for its greater acuity. Would the hand area of the cortex—if we modeled it in rubber and then stood inside and blew gently to get rid of the artificial creases—really resemble a glove? Probably not. Determining the map of the somatosensory cortex has turned out to be a daunting task. The results so far suggest that the predicted shape is just too bizarre; instead, the surface is cut up into manageable pieces as if with scissors, and pasted back together like a quilt so as to approximate a flat surface.

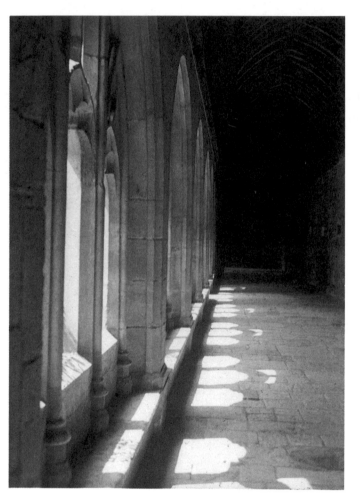 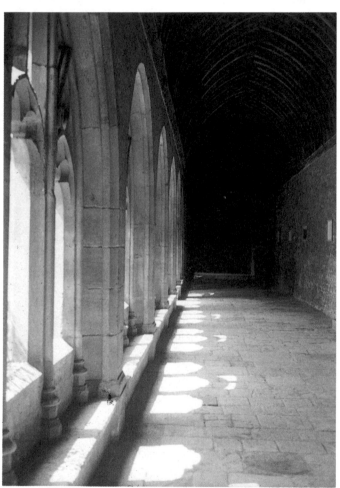

Stereopair of the Cloisters, New College, Oxford. The right photograph was taken, the camera was shifted about 3 inches to the left, and the left photograph was taken.

7

THE CORPUS CALLOSUM
AND STEREOPSIS

The *corpus callosum,* a huge band of myelinated fibers, connects the two cerebral hemispheres. *Stereopsis* is one mechanism for seeing depth and judging distance. Although these two features of the brain and vision are not closely related, a small minority of corpus-callosum fibers do play a small role in stereopsis. The reason for including the two subjects in one chapter is convenience: what I will have to say in both cases relies heavily on the special crossing and lack-of-crossing of optic nerve fibers that occurs at the optic chiasm (see illustration on p. 60), and it is easiest to think about both subjects with those anatomical peculiarities in mind.

THE CORPUS CALLOSUM

The corpus callosum (Latin for "tough body") is by far the largest bundle of nerve fibers in the entire nervous system. Its population has been estimated at 200 million axons—the true number is probably higher, as this estimate was based on light microscopy rather than on electron microscopy— a number to be contrasted to 1.5 million for each optic nerve and 32,000 for the auditory nerve. Its cross-sectional area is about 700 square millimeters, compared with a few square millimeters for the optic nerve. It joins the two cerebral hemispheres, along with a relatively tiny fascicle of fibers called the *anterior commissure,* as shown in the two illustrations on the following pages. The word *commissure* signifies a set of fibers connecting two homologous neural structures on opposite sides of the brain or spinal cord; thus the corpus callosum is sometimes called the great cerebral commissure.

Until about 1950 the function of the corpus callosum was a complete mystery. On rare occasions, the corpus callosum in humans is absent at birth, in a

The corpus callosum is a thick, bent plate of axons near the center of this brain section, made by cutting apart the human cerebral hemispheres and looking at the cut surface.

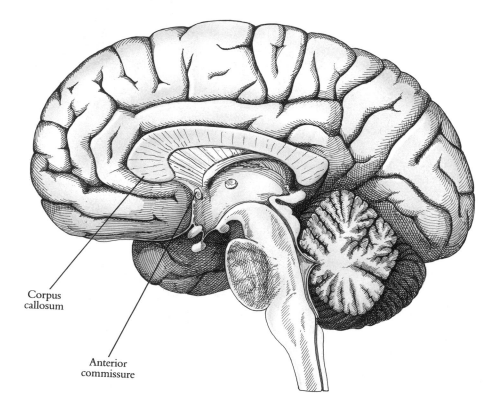

Corpus
callosum

Anterior
commissure

condition called *agenesis of the corpus callosum*. Occasionally it may be completely or partially cut by the neurosurgeon, either to treat epilepsy (thus preventing epileptic discharges that begin in one hemisphere from spreading to the other) or to make it possible to reach a very deep tumor, such as one in the pituitary gland, from above. In none of these cases had neurologists and psychiatrists found any deficiency; someone had even suggested (perhaps not seriously) that the sole function of the corpus callosum was to hold the two cerebral hemispheres together. Until the 1950s we knew little about the detailed connections of the corpus callosum. It clearly connected the two cerebral hemispheres, and on the basis of rather crude neurophysiology it was thought to join precisely corresponding cortical areas on the two sides. Even cells in the striate cortex were assumed to send axons into the corpus callosum to terminate in the exactly corresponding part of the striate cortex on the opposite side.

In 1955 Ronald Myers, a graduate student studying under psychologist Roger Sperry at the University of Chicago, did the first experiment that revealed a function for this immense bundle of fibers. Myers trained cats in a box

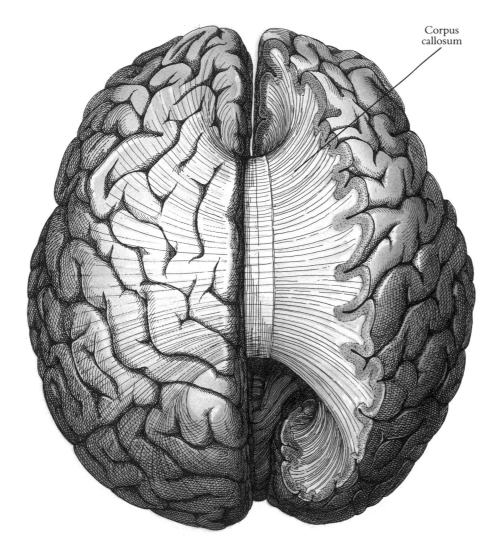

Corpus callosum

Here the brain is seen from above. On the right side an inch or so of the top has been lopped off. We can see the band of the corpus callosum fanning out after crossing, and joining every part of the two hemispheres. (The front of the brain is at the top of the picture.)

containing two side-by-side screens onto which he could project images, for example a circle onto one screen and a square onto the other. He taught a cat to press its nose against the screen with the circle, in preference to the one with the square, by rewarding correct responses with food and punishing mistakes mildly by sounding an unpleasantly loud buzzer and pulling the cat back from the screen gently but firmly. By this method the cat could be brought to a fairly consistent performance in a few thousand trials. (Cats learn slowly; a pigeon will learn a similar task in tens to hundreds of trials, and we humans can learn simply by being told. This seems a bit odd, given that a cat's brain is many times the size of a pigeon's. So much for the sizes of brains.)

Not surprisingly, Myers' cats could master such a task just as fast if one eye was closed by a mask. Again not surprisingly, if a task such as choosing a triangle or a square was learned with the left eye alone and then tested with the right eye alone, performance was just as good. This seems not particularly impressive, since we too can easily do such a task. The reason it is easy must be related to the anatomy. Each hemisphere receives input from both eyes, and as we saw in Chapter 4, a large proportion of cells in area 17 receive input from both eyes. Myers now made things more interesting by surgically cutting the optic chiasm in half, by a fore-and-aft cut in the midline, thus severing the crossing fibers but leaving the uncrossed ones intact—a procedure that takes some surgical skill. Thus the left eye was attached only to the left hemisphere and the right eye to the right hemisphere. The idea now was to teach the cat through the left eye and test it with the right eye: if it performed correctly, the information necessarily would have crossed from the left hemisphere to the right through the only route known, the corpus callosum. Myers did the experiment: he cut the chiasm longitudinally, trained the cat through one eye, and tested it through the other—and the cat still succeeded. Finally, he repeated the experiment in an animal whose chiasm and corpus callosum had both been surgically divided. The cat now failed. Thus he established, at long last, that the callosum actually could do something—although we would hardly suppose that its sole purpose was to allow the few people or animals with divided optic chiasms to perform with one eye after learning a task with the other.

STUDIES OF THE PHYSIOLOGY OF THE CALLOSUM

One of the first neurophysiological examinations of the corpus callosum was made a few years after Myers' experiments by David Whitteridge, then in Edinburgh. Whitteridge realized that for a band of nerve fibers to join homologous, mirror-symmetric parts of area 17 made no sense. No reason could possibly exist for wanting a cell in the left hemisphere, concerned with points somewhere out in the right field of vision, to be connected to a cell on the other side, concerned with points equally far out in the left field. To check this further Whitteridge surgically severed the optic tract on the right side, just behind the optic chiasm, thus detaching the right occipital lobe from the out-

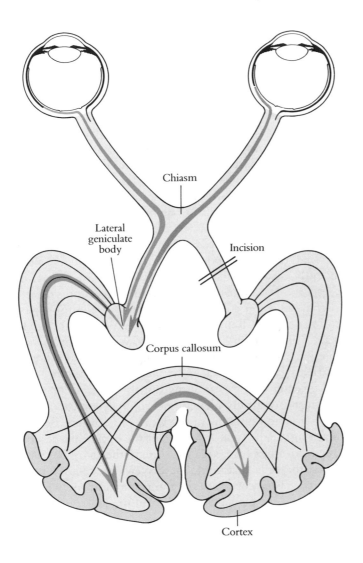

Chiasm

Lateral
geniculate
body

Incision

Corpus callosum

Cortex

In his experiment, Whitteridge cut the right optic tract. For information to get from either eye to the right visual cortex, it now has to go to the left visual cortex and cross in the corpus callosum. Cooling either of these areas blocks the flow of nerve impulses.

side world—except, of course, for any input that area might receive from the left occipital lobe via the corpus callosum, as you can see from the illustration on this page. He then looked for responses by shining light in the eyes and recording from the right hemisphere with wire electrodes placed on the cortical surface. He did record responses, but the electrical waves he observed appeared only at the inner border of area 17, a region that gets its visual input from a long, narrow, vertical strip bisecting the visual field: when he used smaller spots of light, they produced responses only when they were flashed in

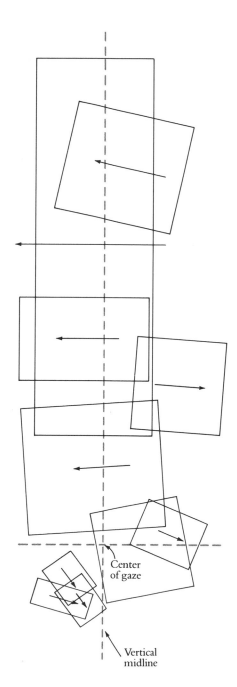

Center
of gaze

Vertical
midline

The receptive fields of fibers in the corpus
callosum lie very close to the vertical midline. The receptive fields here were found
by recording from ten fibers in one cat.

parts of the visual field at or near the vertical midline. Cooling the cortex on
the opposite side, thus temporarily putting it out of commission, abolished the
responses, as did cooling the corpus callosum. Clearly, the corpus callosum
could not be joining all of area 17 on the two sides, but just a small part
subserving the vertical midline of the visual field.

Anatomical experiments had already suggested such a result. Only the parts
of area 17 very close to the border between areas 17 and 18 sent axons across to
the other side, and these seemed to end, for the most part, in area 18, close to
its border with area 17. If we assume that the input the cortex gets from the
geniculates is strictly from contralateral visual fields—left field to right cortex
and right field to left cortex—the presence of corpus-callosum connections
between hemispheres should result in one hemisphere's receiving input from
more than one-half the visual fields: the connections should produce an overlap in the visual-field territories feeding into the two hemispheres. That is, in
fact, what we find. Two electrodes, one in each hemisphere near the 17-18
borders, frequently record cells whose fields overlap by several degrees.

Torsten Wiesel and I soon made microelectrode recordings directly from the
part of the corpus callosum containing visual fibers, the most posterior por-
tion. We found that nearly all the fibers that we could activate by visual stimuli
responded exactly like ordinary cells of area 17, with simple or complex properties, selective for orientation and responding usually to both eyes. They all
had receptive fields lying very close to the vertical midline, either below,
above, or in the center of gaze, as shown in the diagram on this page.

Perhaps the most esthetically pleasing neurophysiological demonstration of
corpus-callosum function came from the work of Giovanni Berlucchi and Gi-
acomo Rizzolatti in Pisa in 1968. Having cut the optic chiasm along the midline, they made recordings from area 17, close to the 17-18 border on the right
side, and looked for cells that could be driven binocularly. Obviously any
binocular cell in the visual cortex on the right side must receive input from the
right eye directly (via the geniculate) and from the left eye by way of the left
hemisphere and corpus callosum. Each binocular receptive field spanned the
vertical midline, with the part to the left responding to the right eye and the
part to the right responding to the left eye. Other properties, including orientation selectivity, were identical, as shown in the illustration on the facing
page.

This result showed clearly that one function of the corpus callosum is to
connect cells so that their fields can span the midline. It therefore cements
together the two halves of the visual world. To imagine this more vividly,
suppose that our cortex had originally been constructed out of one piece instead of being subdivided into two hemispheres; area 17 would then be one
large plate, mapping the entire visual field. Neighboring cells would of course
be richly interconnected, so as to produce the various response properties,
including movement responses and orientation selectivity. Now suppose a dicta-

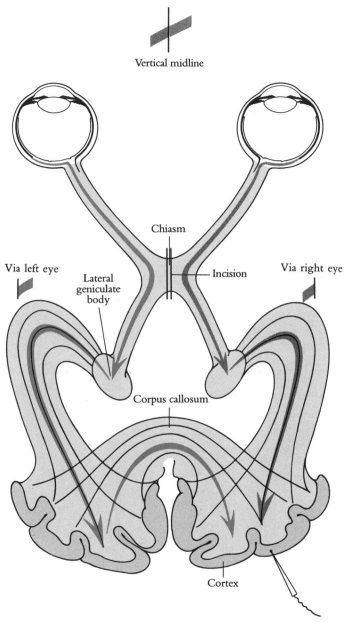

Vertical midline

Chiasm

Via left eye

Via right eye

Lateral geniculate body

Incision

Corpus callosum

Cortex

This experiment by Berlucchi and Rizzolatti beautifully illustrates not only the function of the visual part of the callosum but also the high specificity of its connections between cells of like orientation and bordering receptive fields. Berlucchi and Rizzolatti cut the chiasm of a cat in the midline, so that the left eye supplies only the left hemisphere, with information coming solely from the right field of vision. Similarly, the right eye supplies only the right hemisphere, with information from the left visual field. After making the incision, they recorded from a cell whose receptive field would normally overlap the vertical midline. They found that such a cell's receptive field is split vertically, with the right part supplied through the left eye and the left part through the right eye.

tor (the deity, evolution, or whatever) decides this will no longer do: half the cells must henceforth go to one hemisphere and half to the other. What to do about all those rich connections between the cells that must now be pulled apart? The connections, we suppose, are simply dragged across and form part of the corpus callosum. To avoid delays in having the signals travel so great a distance (in humans, perhaps 5 to 6 inches) we speed conduction by putting a myelin coating on the axons. Of course, in evolution nothing like this ever really happened, since the brain had two hemispheres long before the cerebral cortex evolved.

This experiment of Berlucchi and Rizzolatti provides the most vivid example I know of the remarkable specificity of neural connections. The cell illustrated on page 143, and presumably a million other callosally connected cells like it, derives a single orientation selectivity both through local connections to nearby cells and through connections coming from a region of cortex in the other hemisphere, several inches away, from cells with the same orientation selectivity and immediately adjacent receptive-field positions—to say nothing of all the other matching attributes, such as direction selectivity, end-stopping, and degree of complexity. Every callosally connected cell in the visual cortex must get its input from cells in the opposite hemisphere with exactly matching properties. We have all kinds of evidence for such selective connectivity in the nervous system, but I can think of none that is so beautifully direct.

Visual fibers such as these make up only a small proportion of callosal fibers. In the somatosensory system, anatomical axon-transport studies, similar to the radioactive-amino-acid eye injections described in earlier chapters, show that the corpus callosum similarly connects areas of cortex that are activated by skin or joint receptors near the midline of the body, on the trunk, back, or face, but does not connect regions concerned with the extremities, the feet and hands.

Every cortical area is connected to several or many other cortical areas on the same side. For example, the primary visual cortex is connected to area 18 (visual area 2), to the medial temporal area (MT), to visual area 4, and to one or two others. Often a given area also projects to several areas in the opposite hemisphere through the callosum or, in some few cases, by the anterior commissure. We can therefore view these commissural connections simply as one special kind of cortico-cortico connection. A moment's thought tells us these links must exist: if I tell you that my left hand is cold or that I see something to my left, I am using my cortical speech area, which is located in several small regions in my left hemisphere, to formulate the words. (This *may* not be true, because I am left handed.) But the information concerning my left field of vision or left hand feeds into my right hemisphere: it must therefore cross over to the speech area if I am going to talk about it. The crossing takes place in the corpus callosum. In a series of studies beginning in the early 1960s, Roger Sperry, now at Cal Tech, and his colleagues showed that a human whose corpus callosum had been cut (to treat epilepsy) could no longer talk about events that had entered through the right hemisphere. These subjects provided a mine of new information on various kinds of cortical function, including thought and consciousness. The original papers, which appeared in the journal *Brain,* make fascinating reading and should be fully understandable to anyone reading the present book.

STEREOPSIS

The strategy of judging depth by comparing the images on our two retinas works so well that many of us who are not psychologists or visual physiologists are not aware of the ability. To satisfy yourself of its importance, try driving a car or bicycle, playing tennis, or skiing for even a few minutes with one eye closed. Stereoscopes are out of fashion, though you can still find them in antique shops, but most of us know about 3-D movies, where you have to wear special glasses. Both of these rely on stereopsis.

The image cast on our retinas is two-dimensional, but we look out on a three-dimensional world. To humans and animals it is obviously important to be able to tell how far away things are. Similarly, determining an object's three-dimensional shape means estimating relative depths. To take a simple example, circular objects unless viewed head-on produce elliptical images, but we can generally recognize them as circular with no trouble; and to do that requires a sense of depth.

We judge depth in many ways, some of which are so obvious that they hardly require mention (but I will anyhow). When the size of something is roughly known, as is so for a person, tree, or cat, we can judge its distance—at the risk of being fooled by dwarves, bonsai, or lions. If one object is partly in front of another and blocks its view, we judge the front object as closer. The images of parallel lines like railroad tracks as they go off into the distance draw closer together: this is an example of perspective, a powerful indicator of depth. A bump on a wall that juts out is brighter on top if the light source comes from above (as light sources generally do), and a pit in a surface lit from above is darker in its upper part: if the light is made to come from below, bumps look like pits and pits like bumps. A major clue to depth is *parallax,* the relative motions of near and far objects that is produced when we move our heads from side to side or up and down. Rotating a solid object even through a small angle can make its shape immediately apparent. If we use our lens to focus on a near object, a far one will be out of focus, and by varying the shape of the lens—by changing accommodation (described in Chapters 2 and 6)—we should be able to determine how far an object is. Changing the relative directions of the eyes, adjusting the toeing in or toeing out, will bring the two images of an object together over a narrow range of convergence or divergence. Thus in principle the adjustment of either lens or eye position could tell us an object's distance, and many range finders are based on these principles. Except for the convergence and divergence, all these depth cues need involve only one eye. Stereopsis, perhaps the most important mechanism for assessing depth, depends on the use of the two eyes together. In any scene with depth, our two eyes receive slightly different images. You can satisfy yourself of this

Left: When an observer looks at a point P, the two images of P fall on the foveas F. Q is a point that is judged by the observer to be the same distance away as P. The two images of Q (Q_L and Q_R) are then said to fall on corresponding points. (The surface made up of all points Q, the same apparent distance away as P, is the horopter through P.) *Right:* If Q′ appears closer to the observer than Q, then the images of Q′ (Q'_L and Q'_R) will be farther apart on the retina in a horizontal direction than they would be if they were corresponding points. If Q′ appears farther away, Q'_L and Q'_R will be horizontally displaced toward each other.

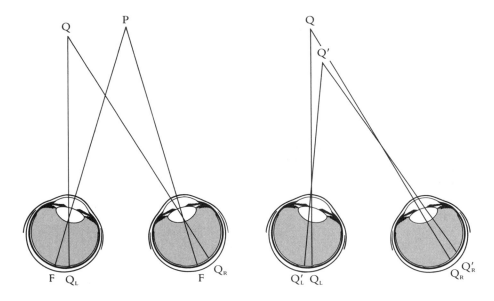

simply by looking straight ahead and moving your head quickly about 4 inches to the right or left or by quickly alternating eyes by opening one and closing the other. If you are facing a flat object, you won't see much difference, but if the scene contains objects at different distances, you will see marked changes. In stereopsis, the brain compares the images of a scene on the two retinas and estimates relative depths with great accuracy.

Suppose an observer fixes his gaze on a point P. This is equivalent to saying that he adjusts his eyes so that the images of P fall on the foveas, F (see the left part of the diagram this page). Now suppose Q is another point in space, which appears to the observer to be the same distance away as P, and suppose Q_L and Q_R are the images of Q on the left and right retinas. Then we say that Q_L and Q_R are *corresponding points* on the two retinas. Obviously, the two foveas are corresponding points; equally obvious, from geometry, a point Q′ judged by the observer to be nearer to him than Q will produce two noncorresponding images Q'_L and Q'_R that are farther apart than they would be if they were corresponding (as shown in the right of the diagram). If you like, they are outwardly displaced relative to each other, compared to the positions corresponding points would occupy. Similarly, a point farther from the observer will give images closer to each other (inwardly displaced) compared to corresponding points. These statements about corresponding points are partly definitions and partly statements based on geometry, but they also involve biology, since they are statements about the judgements of the observer concerning what he considers to be closer or farther than P. All points that, like Q (and of course P), are seen as the same distance away as P are said to lie on the *horopter*, a surface that passes through P and Q and whose exact shape is neither a plane nor a sphere but depends on our estimations of distance, and consequently on our brains. The distance from the foveas F to the images of Q (Q_L and Q_R) are roughly, but not quite, equal. If they *were* always equal, then the horopter would cut the horizontal plane in a circle.

Now suppose we fix our gaze on a point in space and arrange two spotlights that shine a spot on each retina so that the two spots fall on points that are not corresponding but are farther apart than they would be if they were corresponding. We call any such lack of correspondence *disparity*. If the departure from correspondence, or disparity, is in a horizontal direction, is not greater than about 2 degrees (0.6 millimeters on the retina), and has no vertical component greater than a few minutes of arc, what we perceive is a single spot in space, and this spot appears closer than the point we are looking at. If the displacement is inward, the spot will appear farther away. Finally, if the displacement has a vertical component greater than a few minutes of arc or a horizontal component exceeding 2 degrees, the spot will appear double and may or may not appear closer or farther away. This experimental result is the principle of stereopsis, first enunciated in 1838 by Sir Charles Wheatstone, the man who also invented the Wheatstone bridge in electricity.

It seems almost incredible that prior to this discovery, no one seems to have realized that the slight differences in the two pictures projected on our two retinas can lead to a vivid sense of depth. Anyone with a pencil and piece of paper and a few mirrors or prisms or with the ability to cross or uncross his eyes could have demonstrated this in a few minutes. How it escaped Euclid, Archemides, and Newton is hard to imagine. In his paper, Wheatstone describes how Leonardo da Vinci almost discovered it. Leonardo attributed the depth sensation that results from the use of the two eyes to the fact that we see slightly farther around an object on the left with the left eye and on the right with the right eye. As an example of a solid object he chose a sphere— ironically the one object whose shape stays the same when viewed from different directions. Wheatstone remarks that if Leonardo had chosen a cube instead of a sphere he would surely have realized that the two retinal projections are different, and that the differences involve horizontal displacements.

The important biological facts about stereopsis are that the impression of an object being near or far, relative to what we are looking at, comes about if the two images on the retina are horizontally displaced outward or inward relative to each other, as long as the displacement is less than about 2 degrees and as long as vertical displacement is nearly zero. This of course fits the geometry: an object's *being* near or far, relative to some reference distance, produces

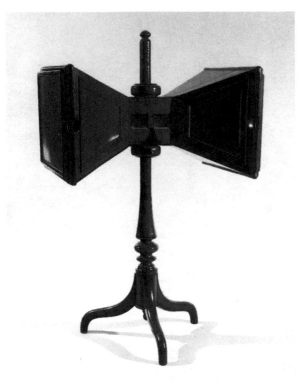

Above: Wheatstone's stereoscope, the original drawing of which is shown to the right.

Right: Wheatstone's diagram of his stereoscope. The observer faced two-45 degree mirrors (A and A′) and saw, superimposed, the two pictures, E through the right eye and E′ through the left. In later, simpler versions, the observer faces the two pictures placed side by side on a screen at a distance apart roughly equal to the distance between the eyes. Two prisms deflect the directions of gaze so that with the eyes aligned as if the observer were looking at the screen, the left eye sees the left picture and the right eye the right picture. You can learn to dispense with the stereoscope by pretending you are looking at a distant object, thus making the two directions of gaze parallel so that the left eye sees the left picture and the right eye the right picture.

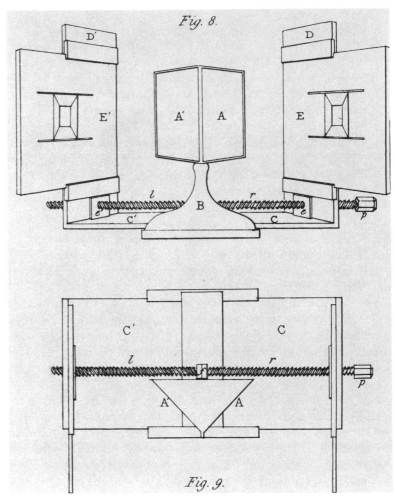

outward or inward displacement of its images on the retinas, without any significant vertical component.

This is the principle of the stereoscope, invented by Wheatstone and for about half a century an object present in almost every household. It is the basis for stereo movies, which we view with special polarized glasses. In the original stereoscope a person looked at two pictures in a box through two mirrors so that each eye saw one picture. To make this easy we often use prisms and focusing lenses. The pictures are identical except for small, relative horizontal displacements, which lead to apparent differences in depth. Anyone can make photographs suitable for a stereoscope by taking a picture of a stationary object, then moving the camera about 2 inches to the left or right and taking another picture.

Not all people have the ability to perceive depth by stereoscopy. You can easily check your stereopsis by using the illustrations on this page: each of the diagrams shows two pictures that together would produce a stereogram for use in an ordinary stereoscope. You can place a copy of these in a stereoscope if you happen to have one, or you can try to look at one with each eye by putting a thin piece of cardboard between them, perpendicular to the plane of the page, and staring, as if you were looking at something far away; you can even learn to cross your eyes, by holding a finger between you and the pictures and adjusting its distance till the two fuse, and then (this is the hard part) examining the fused image without having it break apart. If this works for you, the depth will be reversed relative to the depth you get by the first method.

Even if you don't see the depth, because you have no stereoscope or you can't cross or uncross your eyes, you will still be able to follow the arguments—you just miss the fun.

In the uppermost example, we have a square containing a small circle a little to the right of the center in one member and a little to the left in the other. If you view the figure with both eyes, using the stereoscope or partition method, you should see the circle no longer in the plane of the page but standing out in front of it about an inch or so. Similarly, you should see the second figure as a circle behind the plane of the page. You see the circle in front or behind the page because your retinas are getting exactly the same information they would get if the circle *were* in front or behind.

In 1960 Bela Julesz, at Bell Telephone Laboratories, invented an ingenious, highly useful method for demonstrating stereopsis. The figure on the next page will at first glance seem like a uniformly random mass of tiny triangles—and indeed it is except for the concealed larger triangle in the center part. If you look at it through pieces of colored cellophane, red over one eye and green over the other, you should see the center-triangle region standing out in front

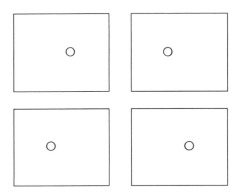

If the upper pair of circles is put in a stereoscope, the circle will stand out in front of the frame. For the lower pair, it will seem to float behind the frame. (You may want to try to superimpose the frames by crossing your eyes or uncrossing them. Most people find uncrossing easier. Placing a thin piece of cardboard between the two images will help. You may at first find this a difficult and disturbing exercise; don't persist very long the first try. With crossed eyes, the upper dot will be farther, the lower one nearer.)

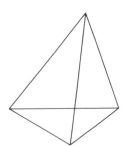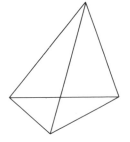

Another stereopair.

To prepare this figure, called an *anaglyph,* Bela Julesz begins by constructing two arrays of randomly placed tiny triangular dots, identical except that (1) one consists of red dots on a white background and the other of green dots on a white background, and (2) over a large triangular region, near the center of the array, all the dots in the green-and-white array are displaced slightly to the left, relative to the corresponding red and white dots. The two arrays are now superimposed with a slight offset, so that the dots themselves do not quite superimpose.

If the figure is viewed through a green cellophane filter, only the red dots are seen; through a red cellophane filter, only the green dots are seen. If you view the figure with green cellophane over the left eye and red over the right, you will see the large triangle standing out about 1 centimeter in front of the page. Reversing the filters (green over the right eye and red over the left) causes the triangle to appear behind.

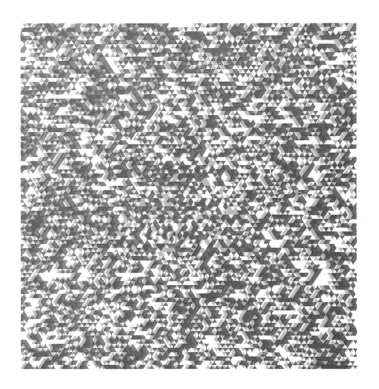

of the page, just as the circle did. (You may, the first time, have to keep looking for a minute or so.) Reversing the cellophane windows will reverse the depth. The usefulness of these Julesz patterns is that you cannot possibly see the triangle standing out in front or receding unless you have intact stereopsis.

To sum up, our ability to see depth depends on five principles:

1. We have many cues to depth, such as occlusion, parallax, rotation of objects, relative size, shadow casting, and perspective. Probably the most important cue is stereopsis.

2. If we fixate on, or look at, a point in space, the images of the point on our two retinas fall on the two foveas. Any point judged to be the same distance away as the point fixated casts its two images on corresponding retinal points.

3. Stereopsis depends on the simple geometric fact that as an object gets closer to us, the two images it casts on the two retinas become outwardly displaced, compared with corresponding points.

4. The central fact of stereopsis—a biological fact learned from testing people—is this: an object whose images fall on corresponding points in the two retinas is perceived as being the same distance away as the point fixated. When the images are outwardly displaced relative to corresponding points, the object is seen as nearer than the fixated point, and when the displacement is inward, the object is seen as farther away.

5. Horizontal displacements greater than about 2 degrees or vertical displacements of over a few minutes of arc lead to double vision.

THE PHYSIOLOGY OF STEREOPSIS

If we want to know how brain cells subserve stereopsis, the simplest question we can ask is whether cells exist whose responses are exquisitely dependent on the relative horizontal positions of images falling on the retinas of the two eyes. We should begin by discussing how cells in the visual pathway respond when the two eyes are stimulated together. We are now talking about cells in area 17 or beyond, because retinal ganglion cells are obviously monocular, and geniculate cells, because of the left-eye, right-eye layering, are for all intents and purposes monocular: they respond to stimulation of either one eye or the other, but not both. In area 17 roughly half the cells are binocular, responding to stimuli in the left eye *and* to stimuli in the right eye. When tested carefully, most of these binocular cells seem not to be greatly concerned with the relative positions of the stimuli in the two eyes. Consider a typical complex cell, which fires continuously if a slit sweeps across its receptive field in either eye. When both eyes are stimulated together, the cell fires at a higher rate than it does to separate eyes, but it generally does not matter much if at any instant the slits in the two retinas fall on exactly the same parts of the two receptive fields. The best responses occur if the slit enters and leaves both eyes' receptive fields at about the same time, but if it enters one a little before or after the other, it doesn't matter very much. A typical curve of response (say, total number of spikes per pass) versus difference in slit position in the two eyes is shown at the top of the next page. The curve is rather flat, clearly indicating that the relative position of the slit in the two eyes is not very important. This kind of cell will fire well to an appropriately oriented slit whether it is at the distance someone is looking, or is nearer or farther away.

Compared with this cell, the cells whose responses are shown on pages 152 (bottom) and 153 are very fussy about the relative positions of the two stimuli and therefore about depth. The first cell (bottom of next page) fires best if the stimuli to the two eyes fall on exactly corresponding parts of the two retinas.

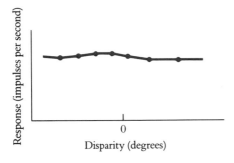

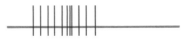

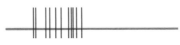

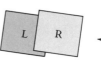

When both eyes are stimulated together by a vertical slit of light moving leftward, an ordinary binocular cell in area 17 will have similar responses to three different relative alignments of the two eyes. Zero disparity means that the two eyes are lined up as they would be if the monkey were looking at the screen onto which the stimuli are being projected. The exact alignment makes little difference in the response of the cell.

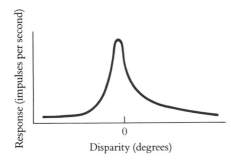

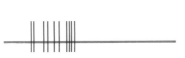

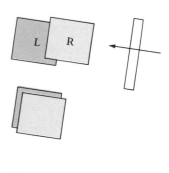

For this "tuned excitatory" cell, it makes a lot of difference whether the stimulus is at the distance the animal is looking, or is nearer or farther away. The cell fires only if the slit is roughly at the distance the animal is looking. In these experiments, the direction of gaze of one eye is varied horizontally with a prism, but bodily moving the screen nearer or farther away would amount to the same thing.

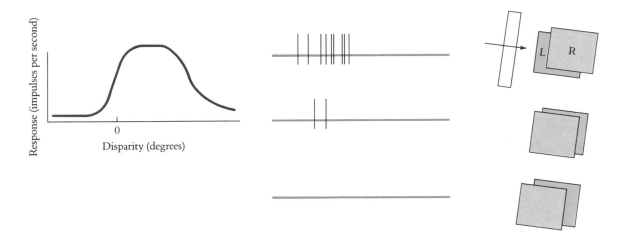

The amount of horizontal malpositioning, or disparity, that can be tolerated before the response disappears is a fraction of the width of the receptive field. It therefore fires if and only if the object is roughly as far away as the distance on which the eyes are fixed. The second cell (top of this page) fires only when the object is farther away than that distance. Still other cells respond only when the stimulus is nearer. As we vary disparity, these two cell types, called *near cells* and *far cells,* both show very rapid changes in responsiveness at or near zero disparity. All three kinds of cells, called *disparity-tuned* cells, have been seen in area 17 of monkeys. It is not yet clear just how common they are or whether they occur in any special layers or in any special relation to ocular-dominance columns. Such cells care very much about the distance of the object from the animal, which translates into the relative positions of the stimulus in the two eyes. Another characteristic feature of these cells is that they fail to respond to either eye alone, or give only weak responses. All these cells have the common characteristic of orientation specificity; in fact, as far as we know, they are like any ordinary upper-layer complex cell, except for their additional fussiness about depth. They respond very well to moving stimuli and are sometimes end stopped.

Gian Poggio at Johns Hopkins Medical School has recorded such cells in area 17 of alert implanted monkeys trained to keep their eyes fixed on a target. In anesthetized monkeys, such cells, although certainly present, seem to be rare in area 17 but are very common in area 18. I would be surprised if an animal or human could assess and compare the distances of objects in a scene stereoscopically if the only cells involved were the three types—tuned excitatory, near, and far—that I have just described. I would have guessed that we would find a whole array of cells for all possible depths. In alert monkeys, Poggio has also seen tuned excitatory cells with peak responses not at zero but

For this cell, a "far" cell, objects closer than the screen evoke little or no response; at about zero disparity (screen distance), a small shift of the screen has a very large influence on the effectiveness of the stimulus. The response rises sharply to a plateau for distances farther away than where the animal is looking. Beyond a certain point the two receptive fields no longer overlap; in effect, the eyes are being stimulated separately. Response then falls to zero.

slightly away from zero, and it thus seems that the cortex may contain cells with all degrees of disparity. Although we still do not know how the brain reconstructs a scene full of objects at various distances (whatever "reconstructs" means), cells such as these seem to represent an early stage in the process.

SOME DIFFICULTIES POSED BY STEREOPSIS

For some years, psychophysicists have recognized the difficult problems that stereopsis poses. Our visual system handles some binocular stimuli in unexpected ways. I could give many examples but will confine myself to two.

We saw in the stereo diagrams on page 149 that displacing two identical images (circles, in that example) inward leads to the sensation "near"; outward, to "far". Now suppose we do both things at once, putting the two circles side by side in each picture. Clearly that *could* give us two circles, one nearer and one farther than the fixation plane. But we could also imagine that the result might simply be two circles lying side by side in the plane of fixation: either situation leads to the same retinal stimuli. In fact, such a pair of stimuli can be seen *only* as two circles side by side, as you will see by fusing the two squares on this page by any of the methods described. Similarly, we can imagine that looking at two diagrams, each consisting of a row of x's, say six of each, side by side, might result in any of a large number of sensations, depending on which x in one eye you pair with which x in the other. In fact, what you get when you view two such diagrams is always six fused x's in the plane of fixation. We don't yet know how the brain resolves the ambiguities and reaches the simplest of all the possible combinations. It is hard to imagine, given the opportunities for ambiguity, how we ever make sense of a scene consisting of a bunch of twigs and branches all at different depths. The physiology, at any rate, tells us that the problem may not be so difficult, since different twigs at different depths are likely to be in different orientations, and as far as we know, stereoscopically tuned cells are always orientation tuned.

The second example of the unpredictability of binocular effects has direct bearing on stereopsis but involves *retinal rivalry,* which we allude to in our discussion of strabismus in Chapter 9. If two very different images are made to fall on the two retinas, very often one will be, as it were, turned off. If you look at the left black-and-white square on the facing page with the left eye and the right one with the right eye, by crossing or uncrossing your eyes or with a stereoscope, you might expect to see a grid, or mesh, like a window screen.

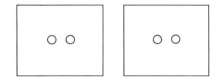

If the figure on page 149 gave you the usual depth effects of a circle standing out in front or floating back behind, the one which combines the two should give *both* a circle in front and one behind. It gives neither, just a pair of circles at the same depth as the frame.

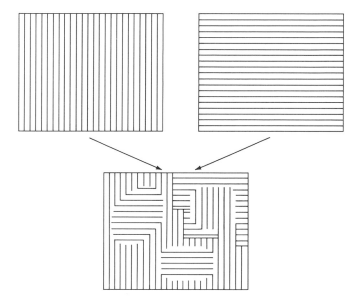

You cannot fuse this pair in the way you can fuse other pairs, such as those on page 149. Instead, you get "retinal rivalry"—a patchwork quilt of vertical and horizontal areas whose borders fade in and out and change position.

Actually, it is virtually impossible to see both sets of orthogonal stripes together. You may see all vertical or all horizontal, with one set coming into view for a few seconds as the other fades, or you may see a kind of patchwork mosaic of the two, in which the patches move and blend in and out from one orientation to the other, as shown by the figure on this page. For some reason the nervous system will not put up with so different simultaneous stimuli in any one part of the visual field—it suppresses one of them. But here we use the word *suppress* as a short way of redescribing the phenomenon: we don't really know how the suppression is accomplished or at what level in the central nervous system it takes place. To me, the patchy quality of the outcome of the battle between the two eyes suggests that the decision takes place rather early in visual processing, conceivably in area 17 or 18. (I am glad I do not have to defend such a guess.)

That we experience retinal rivalry implies that in cases in which the visual system cannot get a sensible result out of the combination of the two sets of inputs from the two eyes—either a single fused flat scene if the images are identical or a scene with depth if the images differ only in small horizontal disparities—it gives up and simply rejects one of the two, either outright, as when you look through a monocular microscope, keeping the other eye open, or in patchy or alternating fashion, as in the example described here. In the case of the microscope, attention surely plays a role, and the neural mechanisms of that role are likewise unknown.

You can see another example of retinal rivalry if you attempt to fuse two patches of different colors, say red and green, instead of vertical and horizontal lines as just described. As I will show in the next chapter, simply mixing red and green light produces the sensation of yellow. On the contrary, when the two colors are presented to separate eyes the result is usually intense rivalry, with red predominating one moment and green the next, and again a tendency for red and green regions to break up into patches that come and go. The rivalry however disappears and one sees yellow if the brightnesses of the patches are carefully adjusted so as to be equal. It seems that color rivalry is produced by differences in brightness rather than differences in hue.

STEREOBLINDNESS

Anyone who is blind in one eye will obviously have no stereopsis. But in the population of people with otherwise normal vision, a surprisingly sizable minority seem to lack stereopsis. If I show stereopairs like the ones on page 149 to a class of 100 students, using polaroids and polarized light, four or five students generally fail to see depth, usually to their surprise, because otherwise they seem to have managed perfectly well. This may seem strange if you have tried the experiment of driving with an eye closed, but it seems that in the absence of stereopsis the other cues to depth—parallax, perspective, depth from movement, occlusion—can in time do very well at compensating. We will see in Chapter 9 that if strabismus, a condition in which the two eyes point in different directions, occurs during infancy, it can lead to the breakdown in connections responsible for binocular interaction in the cortex and, with it, the loss of stereopsis. Since strabismus is common, mild forms of it that were never noticed may account for some cases of stereoblindness. In other cases, people may have a genetic defect in stereopsis, just as they can be genetically color-blind.

Having paired the two topics, corpus callosum and stereopsis, I shouldn't miss the chance to capitalize on what they have in common. You can set yourself the following puzzle: What defect in stereopsis might you expect in someone whose corpus callosum has been severed? The answer is revealed in the illustration on this page.

If you look at point P and consider a point Q, closer than P and falling in the acute angle FPF, the retinal images Q_L and Q_R of Q will fall on opposite sides of the two foveas: Q_L will project to your left hemisphere and Q_R will project to your right hemisphere. This information in the two hemispheres has to connect if the brain is to figure out that Q is closer than P—in other words, if it is to perform stereopsis. The only way it can get together is by the corpus

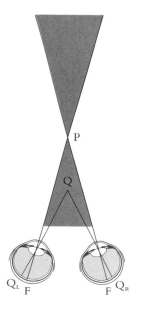

Severing the corpus callosum leads to a loss of stereopsis in the shaded part of a subject's visual world.

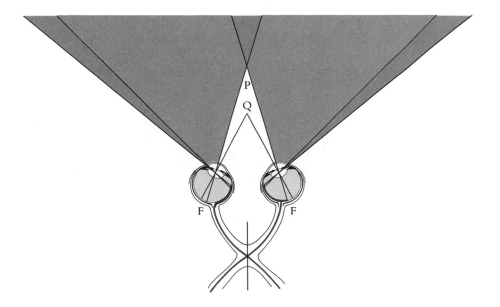

Results of a longitudinal midline section of the optic chiasm: The subject is blind in the two darker wedge-shaped areas at the extreme left and right. Between, in the more lightly shaded areas, stereopsis will be absent, except in the wedge-shaped region beyond P, where there will be no vision at all, and in front of P, where stereopsis will be intact.

callosum. If that path is destroyed, you will be stereoblind in the shaded area. In 1970 Donald Mitchell and Colin Blakemore, at the University of California, Berkeley, tested a subject who had had his corpus callosum cut to relieve epilepsy, and indeed, they found precisely this deficit.

A second, closely related problem is to predict what deficit in stereopsis would result from a midline section of your optic chiasm, such as Ronald Meyers made in cats. This problem is in some ways the opposite of the previous one. From the figure on this page you can see that each eye will be blind in its nasal retina, or its temporal visual field, and so you obviously will have no stereopsis in the lightly shaded areas, where normally it is present. Out beyond this area only one eye can see at a time, so stereopsis is absent even normally; now, however, you will be blind in that region, as indicated by the darker shading. In the area beyond the fixation point, where the blind temporal fields overlap, you will also be blind. Closer than the fixation point, however, your intact visual fields overlap, and stereopsis should be present, provided your corpus callosum is normal. Again, Colin Blakemore found a patient who had fractured his skull as a boy in a bicycle accident and as a consequence apparently sustained a perfect midline section of his optic chiasm. When tested, he proved to have exactly this curious combination of defects and abilities.

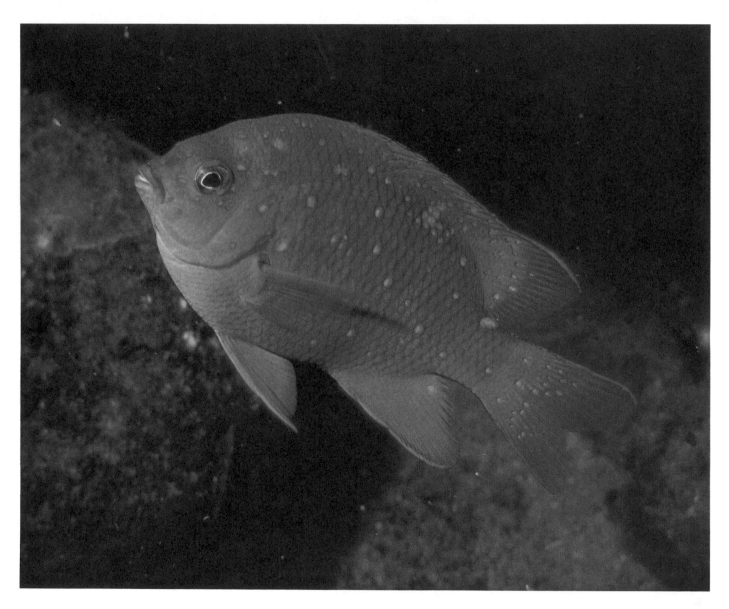

Color serves many purposes in nature, some of which are still mysterious. The blue spots on this Garibaldi fish fade as it grows older, disappearing when it matures. What significance they have for other Garibaldi fish is not known.

8

COLOR VISION

The hundreds of dollars extra that consumers are willing to pay for color TV in preference to black and white must mean that we take our color sense seriously. A complex apparatus in the eye and brain can discriminate the differences in wavelength content of the things we see, and the advantages of this ability to our ancestors are easy to imagine. One advantage must surely have been the ability to defeat the attempts of other animals to camouflage themselves: it is much harder for a hunted animal to blend in with the surroundings if its predator can discriminate the wavelength as well as the intensity of light. Color must also be important in finding plant food: a bright red berry standing out against green foliage is easily found by a monkey, to his obvious advantage and presumably to the plant's, since the seeds pass unharmed through the monkey's digestive tract and are widely scattered. In some animals color is important in reproduction; examples include the bright red coloration of the perineal region of macaque monkeys and the marvelous plumage of many male birds.

In humans, evolutionary pressure to preserve or improve color vision would seem to be relaxing, at least to judge from the 7 or 8 percent of human males who are relatively or completely deficient in color vision but who seem to get along quite well, with their deficit often undiagnosed for years, only to be picked up when they run through red lights. Even those of us who have normal color vision can fully enjoy black-and-white movies, some of which are artistically the best ever made. As I will discuss later, we are all color-blind in dim light.

Among vertebrates, color sense occurs sporadically, probably having been downgraded or even lost and then reinvented many times in the course of evolution. Mammals with poor color vision or none at all include mice, rats, rabbits, cats, dogs, and a species of monkey, the nocturnal owl monkey. Ground squirrels and primates, including humans, apes, and most old world monkeys, all have well-developed color vision. Nocturnal animals whose vision is specialized for dim light seldom have good color vision, which suggests that color discrimination and capabilities for handling dim light are somehow not compatible. Among lower vertebrates, color vision is well developed in many species of fish and birds but is probably absent or poorly developed in reptiles and amphibia. Many insects, including flies and bees, have color vision. We do not know the exact color-handling capabilities of the overwhelming majority of animal species, perhaps because behavioral or physiological tests for color vision are not easy to do.

The subject of color vision, out of all proportion to its biologic importance to man, has occupied an amazing array of brilliant minds, including Newton, Goethe (whose strength seems not to have been science), and Helmholtz. Nevertheless color is still often poorly understood even by artists, physicists, and biologists. The problem starts in childhood, when we are given our first box of paints and then told that yellow, blue, and red are the primary colors and that yellow plus blue equals green. Most of us are then surprised when, in apparent contradiction of that experience, we shine a yellow spot and a blue spot on a screen with a pair of slide projectors, overlap them, and see in the overlapping region a beautiful snow white. The result of mixing paints is mainly a matter of physics; mixing light beams is mainly biology.

In thinking about color, it is useful to keep separate in our minds these different components: physics and biology. The physics that we need to know is limited to a few facts about light waves. The biology consists of psychophysics, a discipline concerned with examining our capabilities as instruments for detecting information from the outside world, and physiology, which examines the detecting instrument, our visual system, by looking inside it to learn how it works. We know a lot about the physics and psychophysics of color, but the physiology is still in a relatively primitive state, largely because the necessary tools have been available for only a few decades.

THE NATURE OF LIGHT

Light consists of particles called photons, each one of which can be regarded as a packet of electromagnetic waves. For a beam of electromagnetic energy to be light, and not X-rays or radio waves, is a matter of the wavelength—the distance from one wave crest to the next—and in the case of light this distance is about 5×10^{-7} meters, or 0.0005 millimeter, or 0.5 micrometer, or 500 nanometers.

Light is defined as what we can see. Our eyes can detect electromagnetic energy at wavelengths between 400 and 700 nanometers. Most light reaching

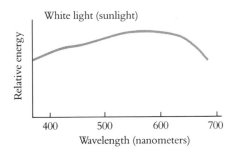

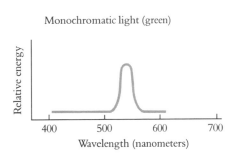

Left: The energy in a beam of light such as sunlight contains a broad distribution of wavelengths, from 400 or less to about 700 nanometers. The gentle peak is a function of the temperature of the source: the hotter the source the more the peak is displaced towards the blue, or short-wavelength, end. *Right:* Monochromatic light is light whose energy is mostly at or near one wavelength. It can be produced with various kinds of filters, with a spectroscope containing a prism or a grating, or with a laser.

our eyes consists of a relatively even mixture of energy at different wavelengths and is loosely called *white light*. To assess the wavelength content of a beam of light we measure how much light energy it contains in each of a series of small intervals, for example, between 400 and 410 nanometers, between 410 and 420 nanometers, and so on, and then draw a graph of energy against wavelength. For light coming from the sun, the graph looks like the left illustration on this page. The shape of the curve is broad and smooth, with no very sudden ups or downs, just a gentle peak around 600 nanometers. Such a broad curve is typical for an incandescent source. The position of the peak depends on the source's temperature: the graph for the sun has its peak around 600 nanometers; for a star hotter than our sun, it would have its peak displaced toward the shorter wavelengths—toward the blue end of the spectrum, or the left in the graph—indicating that a higher proportion of the light is of shorter wavelength. (The artist's idea that reds, oranges, and yellows are warm colors and that blues and greens are cold is related to our emotions and associations, and has nothing to do with the spectral content of incandescent light as related to temperature, or what the physicists call color temperature.)

If by some means we filter white light so as to remove everything but a narrow band of wavelengths, the resulting light is termed *monochromatic* (see the graph at the right on this page).

PIGMENTS

When light hits an object, one of three things can happen: the light can be absorbed and the energy converted to heat, as when the sun warms something; it can pass through the object, as when the sun's rays hit water or glass; or it can be reflected, as in the case of a mirror or any light-colored object, such as a piece of chalk. Often two or all three of these happen; for

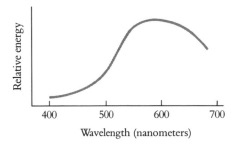

Most colored objects reflect light that is generally richer in some parts of the visible spectrum than in others. The distribution of wavelengths is much broader than that for monochromatic light, however. This graph shows the spectral content of light that would be reflected from a red object, using a broad-band (white) light source.

example, some light may be absorbed and some reflected. For many objects, the relative amount of light absorbed and reflected depends on the light's wavelength. The green leaf of a plant absorbs long- and short-wavelength light and reflects light of middle wavelengths, so that when the sun hits a leaf, the light reflected back will have a pronounced broad peak at middle wavelengths (in the green). A red object will have its peak, likewise broad, in the long wavelengths, as shown in the graph on this page.

An object that absorbs some of the light reaching it and reflects the rest is called a *pigment*. If some wavelengths in the range of visible light are absorbed more than others, the pigment appears to us to be colored. *What* color we see, I should quickly add, is not simply a matter of wavelengths; it depends on wavelength content and on the properties of our visual system. It involves both physics and biology.

VISUAL RECEPTORS

Each rod or cone in our retina contains a pigment that absorbs some wavelengths better than others. The pigments, if we were able to get enough of them to look at, would therefore be colored. A visual pigment has the special property that when it absorbs a photon of light, it changes its molecular shape and at the same time releases energy. The release sets off a chain of chemical events in the cell, described in Chapter 3, leading ultimately to an electrical signal and secretion of chemical transmitter at the synapse. The pigment molecule in its new shape will generally have quite different light-absorbing properties, and if, as is usually the case, it absorbs light less well than it did before the light hit it, we say it is bleached by the light. A complex chemical machinery in the eye then restores the pigment to its original conformation; otherwise, we would soon run out of pigment.

Our retinas contain a mosaic of four types of receptors: rods and three types of cones, as shown in the illustration at the top of the facing page. Each of these four kinds of receptors contains a different pigment. The pigments differ slightly in their chemistry and consequently in their relative ability to absorb light of different wavelengths. Rods are responsible for our ability to see in dim light, a kind of vision that is relatively crude and completely lacks color. Rod pigment, or *rhodopsin*, has a peak sensitivity at about 510 nanometers, in the green part of the spectrum. Rods differ from cones in many ways: they are smaller and have a somewhat different structure; they differ from cones in their relative numbers in different parts of the retina and in the connections they make with subsequent stages in the visual pathway. And finally, in the

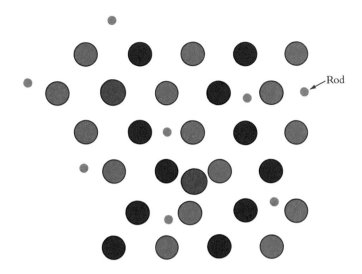

Retinal receptors form a mosaic consisting of rods and the three types of cones. This diagram might represent a part of the retina a few degrees from the fovea, where cones outnumber rods.

light-sensitive pigments they contain, the three types of cones themselves differ from each other and from rods.

The pigments in the three cone types have their peak absorptions at about 430, 530, and 560 nanometers, as shown in the graph on this page; the cones are consequently loosely called "blue", "green", and "red", "loosely" because (1) the names refer to peak sensitivities (which in turn are related to ability to absorb light) rather than to the way the pigments would appear if we were to look at them; (2) monochromatic lights whose wavelengths are 430, 530, and 560 nanometers are not blue, green, and red but violet, blue-green, and yellow-green; and (3) if we were to stimulate cones of just one type, we would see not blue, green, or red but probably violet, green, and yellowish-red instead. However unfortunate the terminology is, it is now widely used, and

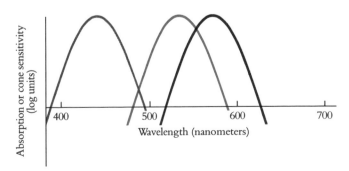

Absorption spectra (or sensitivity curves) differ for the three types of cones. (Spectral-energy curves and absorption curves such as these have their y axes in log units because they operate over such a wide range. The up-and-down position of the x-axis is therefore arbitrary and does not represent zero absorption.)

efforts to change embedded terminology usually fail. To substitute terms such as *long*, *middle*, and *short* would be more correct but would put a burden on those of us not thoroughly familiar with the spectrum.

With peak absorption in the green, the rod pigment, rhodopsin, reflects blue and red and therefore looks purple. Because it is present in large enough amounts in our retinas that chemists can extract it and look at it, it long ago came to be called *visual purple*. Illogical as it is, "visual purple" is named for the appearance of the pigment, whereas the terms for cones, "red", "green", and "blue", refer to their relative sensitivities or abilities to absorb light. Not to realize this can cause great confusion.

The three cones show broad sensitivity curves with much overlap, especially the red and the green cones. Light at 600 nanometers will evoke the greatest response from red cones, those peaking at 560 nanometers, but will likely evoke some response, even if weaker, from the other two cone types. Thus the red-sensitive cone does not respond *only* to long-wavelength, or red, light; it just responds better. The same holds for the other two cones.

So far I have been dealing with physical concepts: the nature of light and pigments, the qualities of the pigments that reflect light to our eyes, and the qualities of the rod and cone pigments that translate the incoming light into electrical signals. It is the brain that interprets these initial signals as colors. In conveying some feel for the subject, I find it easiest to outline the elementary facts about color vision at the outset, leaving aside for the moment the three-century history of how these facts were established or how the brain handles color.

GENERAL COMMENTS ON COLOR

It may be useful to begin by comparing the way our auditory systems and our visual systems deal with wavelength. One system leads to tone and the other to color, but the two are profoundly different. When I play a chord of five notes on the piano, you can easily pick out the individual notes and sing them back to me. The notes don't combine in our brain but preserve their individuality, whereas since Newton we have known that if you mix two or more beams of light of different colors, you cannot say what the components are, just by looking.

A little thought will convince you that color vision has to be an impoverished sense, compared with tone perception. Sound coming to one ear at any instant, consisting of some combination of wavelengths, will influence thousands of receptors in the inner ear, each tuned to a slightly different pitch than the next receptor. If the sound consists of many wavelength components, the information will affect many receptors, all of whose outputs are sent to our brains. The richness of auditory information comes from the brain's ability to analyze such combinations of sounds.

Vision is utterly different. Its information-handling capacity resides largely in the image's being captured by an array of millions receptors, at every instant. We take in the complex scene in a flash. If we wanted in addition to handle wavelength the way the ear does, the retina would need not only to have an array of receptors covering its surface, but to have, say, one thousand receptors for each point on the retina, each one with maximum sensitivity to a different wavelength. But to squeeze in a thousand receptors at each point is physically not possible. Instead, the retina compromises. At each of a very large number of points it has three different receptor types, with three different wavelength sensitivities. Thus with just a small sacrifice in resolution we end up with some rudimentary wavelength-handling ability over most of our retina. We see seven colors, not eighty-eight (both figures should be much higher!), but in a single scene each point of the many thousands will have a color assigned to it. The retina cannot have both the spatial capabilities that it has and also have the wavelength-handling capacity of the auditory system.

The next thing is to get some feel for what it means for our color vision to have three visual receptors. First, you might ask, if a given cone works better at some wavelengths than at others, why not simply measure that cone's output and deduce what the color is? Why not have one cone type, instead of three? It is easy to see why. With one cone, say the red, you wouldn't be able to tell the difference between light at the most effective wavelength, about 560 nanometers, from a brighter light at a less effective wavelength. You need to be able to distinguish variations in brightness from variations in wavelength.

But suppose you have two kinds of cones, with overlapping spectral sensitivities—say, the red cone and the green cone. Now you can determine wavelength simply by *comparing* the outputs of the cones. For short wavelengths, the green cone will fire better; at longer and longer wavelengths, the outputs will become closer and closer to equal; at about 580 nanometers the red surpasses the green, and does progressively better relative to it as wavelengths get still longer. If we subtract the sensitivity curves of the two cones (they are logarithmic curves, so we are really taking quotients), we get a curve that is independent of intensity. So the two cones together now constitute a device that measures wavelength.

Then why are not two receptors all we need to account for the color vision that we have? Two would indeed be enough if all we were concerned with was monochromatic light—if we were willing to give up such things as our ability to discriminate colored light from white light. Our vision is such that no monochromatic light, at any wavelength, looks white. That could not be true if we had only two cone types. In the case of red and green cones, by progressing from short to long wavelengths, we go continuously from stimulating just the green cone to stimulating just the red, through all possible green-to-red response ratios. White light, consisting as it does of a mixture of all wavelengths, has to stimulate the two cones in some ratio. Whatever monochromatic wavelength happens to give that same ratio will thus be indistinguishable from white. This is exactly the situation in a common kind of color blindness in which the person has only two kinds of cones: regardless of which one of the three pigments is missing there is always some wavelength of light that the person cannot distinguish from white. (Such subjects are color defective, but certainly not color-blind.)

To have color vision like ours, we need three and only three cone types. The conclusion that we indeed have just three cone types was first realized by examining the peculiarities of human color vision and then making a set of deductions that are a credit to the human intellect.

We are now in a better position to understand why the rods do not mediate color. At intermediate levels of light intensity, rods and cones can both be functioning, but except in rare and artificial circumstances the nervous system seems not to subtract rod influences from cone influences. The cones are compared with one another; the rods work alone. To satisfy yourself that rods do not mediate color, get up on a dark moonlit night and look around. Although you can see shapes fairly well, colors are completely absent. Given the simplicity of this experiment it is remarkable how few people realize that they do without color vision in dim light.

Whether we see an object as white or colored depends primarily (not entirely) on which of the three cone types are activated. Color is the consequence of unequal stimulation of the three types of cones. Light with a broad spectral curve, as from the sun or a candle, will obviously stimulate all three kinds of cones, perhaps about equally, and the resulting sensation turns out to be lack of color, or "white". If we could stimulate one kind of cone by itself (something that we cannot easily do with light because of the overlap of the absorption curves), the result, as already mentioned, would be vivid color—violet, green, or red, depending on the cone stimulated. That the peak sensitivity of what we call the "red cone" is at a wavelength (560 nanometers) that appears to us greenish-yellow is probably because light at 560 nanometers excites both the green-sensitive cone and the red-sensitive cone, owing to the overlap in the green- and red-cone curves. By using longer wavelength light we can stimulate the red cone, relative to the green one, more effectively.

The graphs on the facing page sum up the color sensations that result when various combinations of cones are activated by light of various wavelength compositions.

The first example and the last two should make it clear that the sensation "white"—the result of approximately equal stimulation of the three cones—

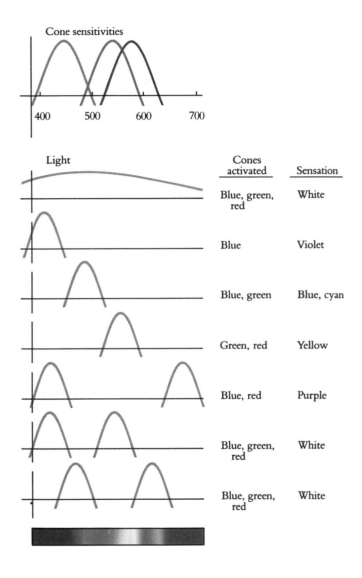

Cone sensitivities

400   500   600   700

Light

Cones activated	Sensation
Blue, green, red	White
Blue	Violet
Blue, green	Blue, cyan
Green, red	Yellow
Blue, red	Purple
Blue, green, red	White
Blue, green, red	White

The top graph, "cone sensitivities", repeats the graph on page 163. The rest of the figure suggests which cones will be activated by various mixtures of colored light and what the resulting sensations will be.

can be brought about in many different ways: by using broad-band light or by using a mixture of narrow-band lights, such as yellow and blue or red and blue-green. Two beams of light are called *complementary* if their wavelength content and intensities are selected so that when mixed they produce the sensation "white". In the last two examples, blue and yellow are complementary, as are red at 640 nanometers and blue-green.

THEORIES OF COLOR VISION

The statements I have made about the relationship between what cones are stimulated and what we see depend on research that began with Newton in 1704 and continues up to the present. The ingenuity of Newton's experiments is hard to exaggerate: in his work on color, he split up white light with a prism; he recombined the light with a second prism, obtaining white again; he made a top consisting of colored segments, which when spun gave white. These discoveries led to the recognition that ordinary light is made up of a continuous mixture of light of different wavelengths.

Gradually, over the eighteenth century, it came to be realized that any color could be obtained by mixtures of light of three wavelengths in the right proportions, provided the wavelengths were far enough apart. The idea that any color could be produced by manipulating three controls (in this case, controls of the intensity of the three lights) was termed *trichromacy*. In 1802 Thomas Young put forward a clear and simple theory to explain trichromacy: he proposed that at each point in the retina there must exist at least three "particles"— tiny light-sensitive structures—sensitive to three colors, red, green, and violet. The long time span between Newton and Young is hard to explain, but various roadblocks, such as yellow and blue paints mixing to produce green, must surely have impeded clear thinking. The definitive experiments that finally proved Young's idea that color must depend on a retinal mosaic of three kinds of detectors was finally confirmed directly and conclusively in 1959, when two groups, George Wald and Paul Brown at Harvard and William Marks, William Dobelle, and Edward MacNichol at Johns Hopkins, examined microscopically the abilities of single cones to absorb light of different wavelengths and found three, and only three, cone types. Meanwhile, scientists had had to do the best they could by less direct means, and they had, in fact, in the course of several centuries arrived at substantially the same result, proving Young's theory that just three types of cones were necessary and estimating their spectral sensitivities. The methods were mainly psychophysical: scientists learned what colors are produced with various mixtures of monochromatic lights, they studied the effects on color vision of selective bleaching with monochromatic lights, and they studied color blindness.

Studies of color mixing are fascinating, partly because the results are so surprising and counterintuitive. No one without prior knowledge would ever guess the various results shown in the illustration on page 167—for example, that two spots, one vivid blue and the other bright yellow, when overlapped would mix to produce a white indistinguishable to the eye from the color of chalk or that spectral green and red would combine to give a yellow almost indistinguishable from monochromatic yellow.

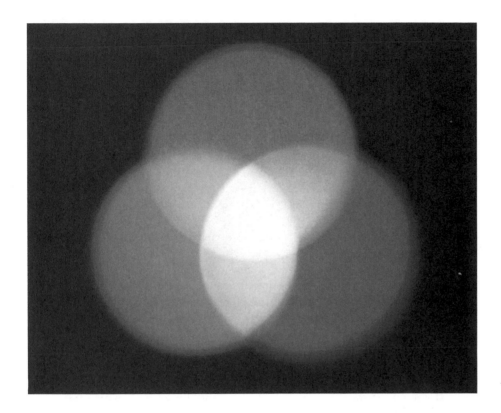

With three slide projectors and three filters, three overlapping spots (red, green, and blue) are projected onto a screen so that they overlap. Red and green give yellow, blue and green give turquoise, red and blue give purple, and all three—red, blue, and green—give white.

Before discussing other theories of color, I should perhaps say more about the variety of colors that theories must account for. What colors are there besides the colors in the rainbow? I can think of three. One kind is the purples, which we don't find in rainbows, but which result from stimulating the red and blue cones, that is, from adding long- and short-wavelength light, or, loosely, red and blue light. If to a mixture of spectral red and blue lights—to purple—we add the right amount of the appropriate green, we get white, and so we say that the green and purple are complementary. You can, if you like, imagine a circular dial that gives all the spectral colors from red through yellow and green to blue and violet, then purples, first bluish-purple and then reddish-purple, and finally back to red. You can even arrange these hues so that complements are opposite each other. The concept of *primary colors* does not even enter this scheme: if we think of primaries in terms of the three receptor types, we have greenish-yellow, green, and violet, shades hardly consistent with the idea of three pure, basic colors. But if by primary we mean three colors from which any other hues can be generated, these three will do, as will any other three that are far enough apart. Thus nothing I have said so far gives any justification for the idea of three unique primary colors.

A second kind of color results from adding white to any spectral color or to purple; we say that the white "washes out" the color, or makes it paler—the technical term is that it *desaturates* it. To match any two colors, we have to make their hues and saturations the same (for example, by selecting the appropriate position on the circle of colors and then adding the right amount of white), and then we need to equate the intensities. Thus we can specify a color by giving the wavelength of the color (or in the case of purple, its complement), the relative content of white, and a single number specifying intensity. A mathematically equivalent option for specifying color is to give three numbers representing the relative effects of the light on the three cone types. Either way, it takes three numbers.

A third kind of color these explanations do not cover is typified by brown. I will come to it later.

Young's theory was adopted and championed by Hermann von Helmholtz and came to be known as the Young-Helmholtz theory. It was Helmholtz, incidentally, who finally explained the phenomenon mentioned at the beginning of this chapter, that mixing yellow and blue paints gives green. You can easily see how this differs from adding yellow and blue light by doing the following experiment, for which you need only two slide projectors and some yellow and blue cellophane. First, put the yellow cellophane over the lens of one projector and the blue over the other and then overlap the projected images. If you adjust the relative intensities, you will get a pure white in the area of overlap. This is the kind of color mixing we have been talking about, and we have said that the white arises because the combined yellow and blue light manages to activate all three of our cones with the same relative effectiveness that broad-band, or white, light does. Now turn off one projector and put both filters in front of the other one, and you will get green. To understand what is happening we need to know that the blue cellophane absorbs long-wavelength light, the yellows and reds, from the white and lets through the rest, which looks blue, and that the yellow filter absorbs mainly blue and lets through the rest, which looks yellow. The diagram on the facing page shows the spectral composition of the light each filter passes. Note that in both cases the light that gets through is far from monochromatic, the yellow light is not narrow-band spectral yellow but a mixture of spectral yellow and shorter wavelengths, greens, and longer wavelengths, oranges and reds. Similarly, the blue is spectral blue plus greens and violet. Why don't we see more than just yellow or just blue? Yellow is the result of equal stimulation of the red and the green cones, with no stimulation of the blue cone; this stimulation can be accomplished with spectral yellow (monochromatic light at 580 nanometers) or with a broader smear of wavelengths, such as we typically get with pig-

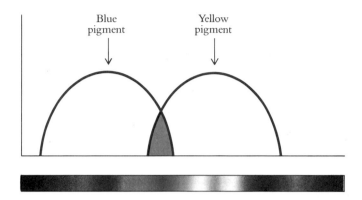

The blue filter passes a fairly broad band of wavelengths centered about 480 nanometers. The yellow filter passes a fairly broad band of wavelengths centered about 580 nanometers. Both together pass only wavelengths common to the two—light at a fairly broad band of wavelengths centered about 530, which gives a green.

ments, as long as the breadth is not so great as to include short wavelengths and thereby stimulate the blue cone. Similarly, as far as our three cones are concerned, spectral blue light has about the same impact as blue plus green plus violet. Now, when we use the two filters, one in front of the other, what we get is what *both* filters let through, namely, just the greens. This is where the graphs shown on this page, for broad-band blue and yellow, overlap. The same thing happens with paints: yellow and blue paints together absorb everything in the light except greens, which are reflected. Note that if we used monochromatic yellow and blue filters in our experiment, putting one in front of the other would result in nothing getting through. The mixing works only because the colors produced by pigments have a broad spectral content.

Why discuss this phenomenon here? I do so partly because it is gratifying to explain the dramatic and startling result of mixing yellow and blue paint to get green, and the even more startling result—because it is so unfamiliar to most people—of mixing yellow and blue light to get *white*. (In a chapter on color theory in a book on weaving, I found the statement that if you mix yellow and blue threads, as in warp and weft, you get green. What you do get is gray—for biological reasons.) The artificial results of mixing paints is doubtless what has led to the idea of "primary colors," such as red, yellow, and blue. If any special set of colors deserves to be called primary, it is the set of red, blue, yellow, and green. As we will see in the section on Hering's color theory, what justification all four have as candidates for primaries has little to do with the three cones and much to do with the subsequent wiring in the retina and brain.

THE GENETICS OF VISUAL PIGMENTS

In the early 1980s Jeremy Nathans, while still an MD-Ph D student at Stanford, managed to clone the genes for the protein portions of human rhodopsin and all three cone pigments. He found that all four pigments show strong homologies in their amino acid sequences: the genes for the red and green pigments, which lie on the X, or sex, chromosome, are virtually identical—the amino acid sequences of the proteins show 96 percent identity—whereas the genes that code for the blue pigment, on chromosome 7, and for rhodopsin, on chromosome 3, show much larger differences, from each other and from the red and green genes. Presumably, some time in the distant past, a primordial visual pigment gave rise to rhodopsin, the blue pigment, and the common precursor of the red and green pigments. At a much more recent time the X-chromosome genes for the red and green pigments arose from this precursor by a process of duplication. Possibly this occurred after the time of separation of the African and South American continents, 30 to 40 million years ago, since old world primates all exhibit this duplication of cone pigment genes on the X-chromosome, whereas new world primates do not.

Cloning the genes has led to a spectacular improvement in our understanding of the various forms of color blindness. It had long been known that most forms of color-vision deficiency are caused by the absence or abnormality of one or more of the three cone pigments. The most frequent abnormalities occur in the red and green pigments and affect about 8 percent of males. Because of the wide range of these abnormalities the subject is complex, but given our molecular-level understanding, it is fortunately no longer bewildering.

Very rarely, destruction to certain cortical areas can cause color blindness. Most often this occurs as the result of a stroke.

THE HERING THEORY

In the second half of the nineteenth century, a second school of thought arose parallel to, but until recently seemingly irreconcilable with, the Young-Helmholtz color theory. Ewald Hering (1834–1918) interpreted the results of color mixing by proposing the existence, in the eye, brain, or both, of three *opponent processes*, one for red-green sensation, one for yellow-blue, and a third, qualitatively different from the first two, for black-white. Hering was impressed by the nonexistence of any colors—and the impossibility of even imagining any colors—that could be described as yellowish-blue or reddish-green and by the apparent mutual canceling of blue and yellow or of red and green when they are added together in the right proportions, with complete elimination of hue—that is, with the production of white. Hering envisioned the red-green and yellow-blue processes as independent, in that blue and red do add to give bluish-red, or purple; similarly red added to yellow gives orange; green added to blue gives bluish-green; green and yellow gives greenish-yellow. In Hering's system, yellow, blue, red, and green could be thought of as "primary" colors. Anyone looking at orange can imagine it to be the result of mixing red and yellow, but no one looking at red or blue would see it as the result of mixing any other colors. (The feeling that some people have that green looks like yellow added to blue is probably related to their childhood experience with paint boxes.) Hering's notions of red-green and yellow-blue processes seemed to many to be disconcertingly dependent on intuitive impressions about color, but it is surprising how good the agreement is among people asked to select the point on the spectrum where blue is represented, untainted by any subjective trace of green or yellow. The same is so for yellow and green. With red, subjects again agree, this time insisting that some violet by added to counteract the slight yellowish appearance of long-wavelength light. (It is this subjective red that when added to green gives white; ordinary (spectral) red added to green gives yellow.)

We can think of Hering's yellow-blue and red-green processes as separate channels in the nervous system, whose outputs can be represented as two meters, like old-fashioned voltmeters, with the indicator of one meter swinging to the left of zero to register yellow and to the right to register blue and the other meter doing the same for red versus green. The color of an object can then be described in terms of the two readings. Hering's third antagonistic process (you can think of it as a third voltmeter) registered black versus white. He realized that black and gray are not produced simply by absence of light coming from an object or surface but arise when and only when the light from the object is less than the average of the light coming from the surrounding regions. White arises only when the surround is darker and when no hue is present. (I have already discussed this in Chapter 3, with examples such as the turned-off television set.) In Hering's theory, the black-white process requires a *spatial* comparison, or subtraction of reflectances, whereas his yellow-blue and red-green processes represent something occurring in one particular place in the visual field, without regard to the surrounds. (Hering was certainly aware that neighboring colors interact, but his color theory as enunciated in his latest work does not encompass those phenomena.) We have already seen that black versus white is indeed represented in the retina and brain by spatially opponent excitatory and inhibitory (on versus off) processes that are literally antagonistic.

Hering's theory could account not only for all hues and levels of saturation, but also for colors such as brown and olive green, which are not only absent from any rainbow, but cannot be produced in any of the classical psychophysical color-mixing procedures, in which we shine spots of light on a dark screen with a slide projector. We get brown only when a yellow or orange spot of light is surrounded by light that on the average is brighter. Take any brown and exclude all the surround by looking at it through a tube, a black piece of rolled up paper, and you will see yellow or orange. We can regard brown as a mixture of black—which is obtainable only by spatial contrasts—and orange or yellow. In Hering's terms, at least two of the systems are at work, the black-white and the yellow-blue.

Hering's theory of three opponent systems, for red-green, yellow-blue, and black-white, was regarded in his time and for the next half-century as rivaling and contradicting the Young-Helmholtz three-pigment (red, green, and blue) theory: the proponents of each were usually strongly partisan and often emotional. Physicists generally sided with the Young-Helmholtz camp, perhaps because their hearts were warmed by the quantitative arguments—by such things as linear simultaneous equations—and turned or cooled off by arguments about purity of colors. Psychologists often sided with Hering, perhaps because they had experience with a wider variety of psychophysical phenomena. Hering's theory seemed to be arguing for either four receptor types (red, green, yellow, and blue) or worse, for three (one subserving black-white, one yellow-blue, and one red-green), all in the face of mounting evidence for the original Young hypothesis. In retrospect, as the contemporary psychophysicists Leo Hurvich and Dorothea Jameson have pointed out, it seems that one difficulty many people had with the Hering theory was the lack, until the 1950s, of any direct physiological evidence for inhibitory mechanisms in sensory systems. Such evidence became available only a half-century later, with single-unit recordings.

By imagining the voltmeters to be measuring positive to the right and negative to the left, you can see why Hering's work suggested inhibitory mechanisms. In a sense, the colors yellow and blue are mutually antagonistic; together they cancel each other, and if the red-green system also reads zero, we have no color. Hering in some ways was fifty years ahead of his time. As has happened before in science, two theories, for decades seemingly irreconcilable, both turned out to be correct. In the late 1800s, nobody could have guessed that at one and the same time the Young-Helmholtz notions of color would turn out to be correct at the receptor level, whereas Hering's ideas of opponent processes would be correct for subsequent stages in the visual path. It is now clear that the two formulations are not mutually exclusive: both propose a three-variable system: the three cones in the Young-Helmholtz and the three meters, or processes, in the Hering theory. What amazes us today is that with so little to go on, Hering's formulation turned out to describe cell-level central-nervous-system color mechanisms so well. Nevertheless, color-vision experts are still polarized into those who feel Hering was a prophet and those who feel that his theories represent a fortuitous fluke. To the extent that I am slightly to the Hering side of center, I will doubtless make enemies of all the experts.

COLOR AND
THE SPATIAL VARIABLE

We saw in Chapter 3 that an object's whiteness, blackness, or grayness depends on the light that the object reflects from some source, relative to the light reflected by the other objects in the scene, and that broad-band cells at an early stage in the visual pathway—retinal ganglion cells or geniculate cells—can go far to account for this perception of black and white and gray: they make just this kind of comparison with their center-surround receptive fields. This is surely Hering's third, spatially opponent black-white process. That the spatial variable is also important for color first began to be appreciated a century ago. It was tackled analytically only in the last few decades, notably by psychophysicists such as Leo Hurvich and Dorothea Jameson, Deane Judd, and Edwin Land. Land, with a consuming interest in light and photography, was naturally impressed by a camera's failure to compensate for differences in light sources. If a film is balanced so that a picture of a white shirt looks white in tungsten light, the same shirt under a blue sky will be light blue; if the film is manufactured to work in natural light, the shirt under tungsten light will be pink. To take a good color picture we have to take into account not only light intensity, but also the spectral content of the light source, whether it is bluish or reddish. If we have that information, we can set the shutter speed and the lens opening to take care of the intensity and select the film or filters to take care of color balance. Unlike the camera, our visual system does all this automatically, and it solves the problem so well that we are generally not aware that a problem exists. A white shirt thus continues to look white in spite of large shifts in the spectral content of the light source, as in going from overhead sun to setting sun, to tungsten light, or to fluorescent light. The same constancy holds for colored objects, and the phenomenon, as applied to color and white, is called *color constancy*. Even though color constancy had been recognized for many years, Land's demonstrations in the 1950s came as a great surprise, even to neurophysiologists, physicists, and most psychologists.

What were these demonstrations? In a typical experiment, a patchwork of rectangular papers of various colors resembling a Mondrian painting is illuminated with three slide projectors, one equipped with a red, the second with a green, the third with a blue filter. Each projector is powered by a variable electric source so that its light can be adjusted over a wide range of intensities. The rest of the room must be completely dark. With all three projectors set at moderate intensities, the colors look much as they do in daylight. The surprising thing is that the exact settings do not seem to matter. Suppose we select a green patch and with a photometer precisely measure the intensity of the light coming from that patch when only one projector is turned on. We then repeat

In many of his experiments Edwin Land used a Mondrian-like patchwork of colored papers. The experiments were designed to prove that the colors remain remarkably constant despite marked variations in the relative intensities of the red, green, and blue lights used to illuminate the display.

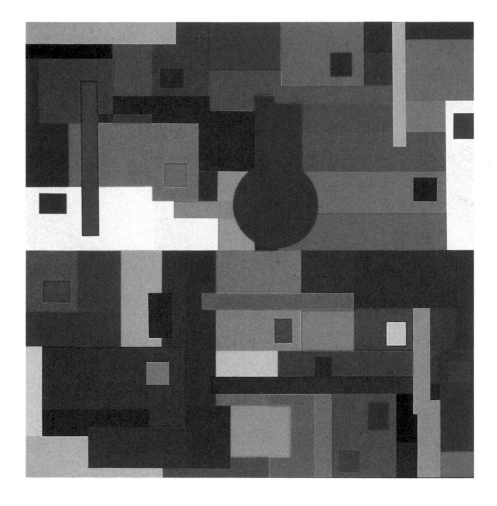

the measurement, first with the second projector and then with the third. That gives us three numbers, representing the light coming to us when we turn on all three projectors. Now we select a different patch, say orange, and readjust each projector's intensity in turn so that the readings we now get from the orange patch are the same as those we got before from the green one. Thus with the three projectors turned on, the composition of light now coming from the orange patch is identical to the composition of light that a moment ago came from the green. What do we expect to see? Naively, we would expect the orange patch to look green. But it still looks orange—indeed, its color has not changed at all. We can repeat this experiment with any two patches. The conclusion is that it doesn't much matter at what intensities the three projectors are set, as long as some light comes from each. In a vivid example of color constancy, we see that twisting the intensity dials for the three projectors to almost any position makes very little difference in the colors of the patches.

Such experiments showed convincingly that the sensation produced in one part of the visual field depends on the light coming from that place *and* on the light coming from everywhere else in the visual field. Otherwise, how could the same light composition give rise at one time to green and at another to orange? The principle that applies in the domain of black, white, and gray, stated so clearly by Hering, thus applies to color as well. For color, we have an opponency not only locally, in red versus green and yellow versus blue, but also spatially: center red-greenness versus surround red-greenness, and the same opponency for yellow-blueness.

In 1985, in Land's laboratory, David Ingle managed to train goldfish to swim to a patch of some preassigned color in an underwater Mondrian display. He found that a fish goes to the same color, say blue, regardless of wavelength content: it selects a blue patch, as we do, even when the light from it is identical in composition to the light that, in a previous trial and under a different light source, came from a yellow patch, which the fish had rejected. Thus the fish, too, selects the patch for its color, not for the wavelength con-

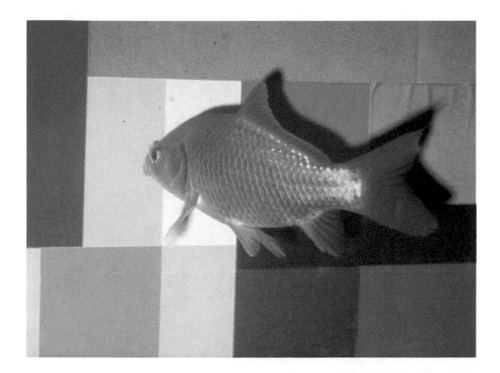

In David Ingle's experiment, a goldfish has been trained to swim to a patch of a given color for a reward—a piece of liver. It swims to the green patch regardless of the exact setting of the three projectors' intensities. The behavior is strikingly similar to the perceptual result in humans.

tent of the light it reflects. This means that the phenomenon of color constancy cannot be regarded as some kind of embellishment recently added by evolution to the color sense of certain higher mammals like ourselves; finding it in a fish suggests that it is a primitive, very basic aspect of color vision. It would be fascinating (and fairly easy) to test and see whether insects with color vision also have the same capability. I would guess that they do.

Land and his group (among others, John McCann, Nigel Daw, Michael Burns, and Hollis Perry) have developed several procedures for predicting the color of an object, given the spectral-energy content of light from each point in the visual field but given no information on the light source. The computation amounts to taking, for each of the three separate projectors, the ratio of the light coming from the spot whose color is to be predicted to the average light coming from the surround. (How much surround should be included has varied in different versions of the theory: in Land's most recent version, the surround effects are assumed to fall off with distance.) The resulting triplet of three numbers—the ratios taken with each projector—uniquely defines the color at that spot. Any color can thus be thought of as corresponding to a point in three-dimensional space whose coordinate axes are the three ratios, taken with red light, green light, and blue light. To make the formulation as realistic as possible, the three lights are chosen to match the spectral sensitivities of the three human cone types.

That color can be so computed predicts color constancy because what counts for each projector are the *ratios* of light from one region to light from the average surround. The exact intensity settings of the projectors no longer matter: the only stipulation is that we have to have *some* light from each projector; otherwise no ratio can be taken. One consequence of all this is that to have color at all, we need to have variation in the wavelength content of light across the visual field. We require color borders for color, just as we require luminance borders for black and white. You can easily satisfy yourself that this is true, again using two slide projectors. With a red filter (red cellophane works well) in front of one of the projectors, illuminate any set of objects. My favorite is a white or yellow shirt and a bright red tie. When so lit, neither the shirt nor the tie looks convincingly red: both look pinkish and washed out. Now you illuminate the same combination with the second projector, which is covered with blue cellophane. The shirt looks a washed-out, sickly blue, and the tie looks black: it's a red tie, and red objects don't reflect short wavelengths. Go back to the red projector, confirming that with it alone, the tie doesn't look especially red. Now add in the blue one. You know that in adding the blue light, you will not get anything more back from the tie—you have just demonstrated that—but when you turn on the blue projector, the red tie suddenly blazes forth with a good bright red. This will convince you that what makes the tie red is not just the light coming to you from the tie.

Experiments with stabilized color borders are consistent with the idea that differences across borders are necessary for color to be seen at all. Alfred Yarbus, whose name came up in the context of eye movements in Chapter 4, showed in 1962 that if you look at a blue patch surrounded by a red background, stabilizing the border of the patch on the retina will cause it to disappear: the blue melts away, and all you see is the red background. Stabilizing the borders on the retina apparently renders them ineffective, and without them, we have no color.

These psychophysical demonstrations that differences in the spectral content of light across the visual field are necessary to perceive color suggest that in our retinas or brains we should find cells sensitive to such borders. The argument is similar to the one we made in Chapter 4, about the perception of black or white objects (such as kidney beans). If at some stage in our visual path color is signaled entirely at color-contrast borders, cells whose receptive fields are entirely within areas of uniform color will be idle. The result is economy in handling the information. We thus find ourselves with two advantages to having color signaled at borders: first, color is unchanged despite changes in the light source, so that our vision tells us about properties of the objects we view, uncontaminated by information about the light source; second, the information handling is economical. Now we can ask why the system evolved the way it did. Are we to argue that the need for color constancy led to the system's evolving and that an unexpected bonus was the economy—or the reverse, that economy was paramount and the color constancy a bonus? Some would argue that the economy argument is more compelling: evolution can hardly have anticipated tungsten or fluorescent lights, and until the advent of supersuds, our shirts were not all that white anyway.

THE PHYSIOLOGY OF COLOR VISION: EARLY RESULTS

The first cell-level physiological information came 250 years after Newton from the studies of the Swedish-Finnish-Venezuelan physiologist Gunnar Svaetichin, who in 1956 recorded intracellularly in teleost fish from what he thought were cones but turned out later to be horizontal cells. These cells responded with slow potentials only (no action potentials) when light was directed on the retina. He found three types of cells, as illustrated on this page: the first, which he called L cells, were hyperpolarized by light stimulation regardless of the light's wavelength composition; the second, called r-g cells,

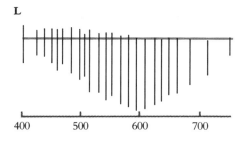

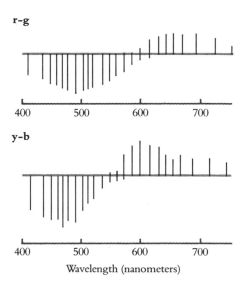

Gunnar Svaetichin and Edward MacNichol recorded the responses to color of horizontal cells in the teleost fish. Deflections pointing downward from the gray line indicate hyperpolarization; those pointing upward indicate depolarization.

were hyperpolarized by short wavelengths, with a maximum response to green light, and depolarized by long wavelengths, with a maximum response to red; the third, which with Hering in mind he called y-b cells, responded like r-g cells but with maximal hyperpolarization to blue and maximal depolarization to yellow. For r-g and y-b cells, white light gave only weak and transient responses, as would be expected from white's broad spectral energy content. Moreover, for both types of cell, which we can call *opponent-color cells*, some intermediate wavelength of light, the *crossover point*, failed to evoke a response. Because these cells react to colored light but not to white light, they are probably concerned with the sensation of color.

In 1958, Russell De Valois (rhymes with *hoi polloi*) and his colleagues recorded responses strikingly similar to Svaetichin's from cells in the lateral geniculate body of macaque monkeys. De Valois had previously shown by behavioral testing that color vision in macaque monkeys is almost identical to color vision in humans; for example, the amounts of two colored lights that have to be combined to match a third light are almost identical in the two species. It is therefore likely that macaques and humans have similar machinery in the early stages of their visual pathways, and we are probably justified in comparing human color psychophysics with macaque physiology. De Valois found many geniculate cells that were activated by diffuse monochromatic light at wavelengths ranging from one end of the spectrum to a crossover point, where there was no response, and were suppressed by light over a second range of wavelengths from the crossover point to the other end. Again the analogy to Hering's color processes was compelling: De Valois found opponent-color cells of two types, red-green and yellow-blue; for each type, combining two lights whose wavelengths were on opposite sides of some crossover point led to mutual cancellation of responses, just as, perceptually, adding blue to yellow or adding green to red produced white. De Valois' results were especially reminiscent of Hering's formulations in that his two classes of color cells had response maxima and crossover points in just the appropriate places along the spectrum for one group to be judging the yellow-blueness of the light and the other, red-greenness.

The next step was to look at the receptive fields of these cells by using small spots of colored light, as Torsten Wiesel and I did in 1966, instead of diffuse light. For most of De Valois' opponent-color cells, the receptive fields had a surprising organization, one that still puzzles us. The cells, like Kuffler's in the cat, had fields divided into antagonistic centers and surrounds; the center could be "on" or "off". In a typical example, the field center is fed exclusively by red cones and the inhibitory surround exclusively by green cones. Consequently, with red light both a small spot and a large spot give brisk responses, because the center is selectively sensitive to long-wavelength light and the surround virtually insensitive; with short-wavelength light, small spots give little or no

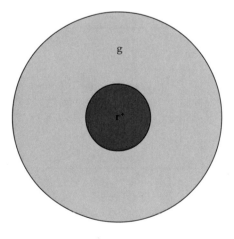

In a typical type 1 receptive field, the center receives excitatory input from red cones; the surround, inhibitory input from green cones.

response and large spots produce strong inhibition with off responses. With white light, containing short and long wavelengths, small spots evoke on responses and large spots produce no response.

Although our first impression was that such a cell must be getting input from red cones in the center region and green cones in the surround, it now seems probable that the total receptive field is a combination of two overlapping processes, as illustrated in the figure on this page. Both the red cones and the green cones feed in from a fairly wide circular area, in numbers that are maximal in the center and fall off with distance from the center. In the center, the red cones strongly predominate, and with distance their effects fall off much more rapidly than those of the green cones. A long-wavelength small spot shining in the center will consequently be a very powerful stimulus to the red system; even if it also stimulates green cones, the number, relative to the total number of green cones feeding in, will be too small to give the red system any competition. The same argument applies to the center-surround cells described in Chapter 3, whose receptive fields similarly must consist of two opponent circular overlapping areas having different-shaped sensitivity-versus-position curves. Thus the surround is probably not annular, or donut shaped, as was originally supposed, but filled. With these opponent-color cells in monkeys, it is supposed—without evidence so far—that the surrounds represent the contributions of horizontal cells.

The responses to diffuse light—in this case, on to red, off to blue or green, and no response to white—make it clear that such a cell must be registering information about color. But the responses to appropriate white borders and the lack of response to diffuse light make it clear that the cell is also concerned with black-and-white shapes. We call these center-surround color-opponent cells "type 1".

The lateral geniculate body of the monkey, we recall from Chapter 4, consists of six layers, the upper four heavily populated with small cells and the lower two sparsely populated with large cells. We find cells of the type just described in the upper, or parvocellular, layers. Type 1 cells differ one from the next in the types of cone that feed the center and surround systems and in the nature of the center, whether it is excitatory or inhibitory. We can designate the example in the diagram on the facing page as "r^+g^-". Of the possible subtypes of cells that receive input from these two cone types, we find all four: r^+g^-, r^-g^+, g^+r^-, g^-r^+. A second group of cells receives input from the blue cone, supplying the center, and from a combination of red and green cones (or perhaps just the green cone), supplying the surround. We call these "blue-yellow", with "yellow" a shorthand way of saying "red-plus-green".

We find two other types of cells in the four dorsal layers. Type 2 cells make up about 10 percent of the population and have receptive fields consisting of a center only. Throughout this center, we find red-green opponency in some

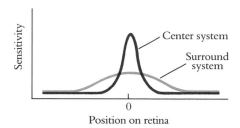

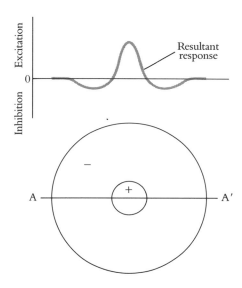

These graphs plot the sensitivity of a cell (measured, for example, by the response to a constant very small spot of light) against retinal position along a line AA' passing through the receptive-field center. For an r^+ center–g^- surround cell, a small red spot gives a narrow curve and a small green spot, a much broader one. The lower graph plots the responses to light such as white or yellow that stimulates both of the opponent systems, so that the two systems subtract. Thus the red cones dominate in the center, which gives on responses, whereas the green cones dominate in the surround, which yields off responses.

cells, blue-yellow in others. The centers of these type 2 cells tend to be large, several times larger than the centers of type 1 cells. The other 15 percent or so of cells in the four upper geniculate layers, and all the cells in the two lower (magnocellular) layers, are center-surround but show no such color preferences; it is as if their field centers and surrounds received the same relative contributions from the three cone types. We refer to these cells as *broad-band*, and in the upper layers we call them type 3 cells.

All these findings are remarkably compatible with Hering's model: we have two classes of color-opponent cells, one red-green, the other yellow-blue, and a third showing no color opponency at all but a broad-band spatial opponency instead. What seemed not to fit any theory was the spatial organization of the opponent-color, or type 1 cells. You might think, at first glance, that this organization would have something to do with color contrast, with the tendency for one color, say blue, to look more vivid if surrounded by another, say green, or for a gray piece of paper to look yellowish if surrounded by blue. But a moment's thought will convince you that type 1 cells can hardly be useful for that kind of color contrast: the r^+ center–g^- surround cell just described, far from being strongly excited by a red spot surrounded by green, gives little or no response, because one effect cancels the other—the reverse of what would seem to be required for color contrast.

What we can say of type 1 cells is that they are likely to play an important part in high-precision form perception, given their tiny field centers and their responsiveness to black-and-white contours. As we saw in Chapter 6, we have several ways to measure visual acuity, the ability of our visual system to discriminate small objects; these include the smallest separation between two dots that can just be discriminated and the smallest detectable gap in a circle (called the Landolt C). Acuity measured in either of these ways turns out, for the fovea, to be about 0.5 minute of arc, or about 1 millimeter at a distance of 8 meters. This corresponds well with the distance between two cones in the fovea. Type 1 geniculate cells that get their input from near the fovea have receptive-field centers as small as about 2 minutes of arc in diameter. It seems likely that in the fovea one cone only contributes to a field center. So we find a reasonable fit between acuity and smallest field-center sizes of lateral geniculate cells.

The ventral pair of geniculate layers differs from the dorsal four in being made up entirely of cells whose field centers are broad-band. The cells do show a curious form of color opponency that no one understands and that I will say no more about. Most people assume that these cells are color-blind. Their field centers are several times larger than centers of parvocellular cells, and they differ in several other interesting ways. We presently suspect that these cells feed into parts of the brain that subserve depth and movement perception. To elaborate further would take us far from color and require another book.

Most of the cells I have been describing for the lateral geniculate have also been observed in the retina. They are more conveniently segregated in the geniculate and are easier to study there. We do not know what the geniculate contributes to the analysis of visual information in the monkey, besides its obvious function of handing on to the cortex the information it receives from the eyes.

THE NEURAL BASIS OF COLOR CONSTANCY

Since type 1 cells in the lateral geniculate body seem not to be geared to make color-spatial comparisons, we probably have to look beyond the retina and geniculate. To test the idea that such computations might go on in the cortex, Land's group and Margaret Livingstone and I examined a man who had had his corpus callosum severed surgically to treat epilepsy. Spatial-color interactions did not take place across the visual-field midline, that is, the color of a spot just to the left of the point at which the subject was looking was not affected by drastic changes in the colors in the right visual field, whereas normal subjects observed marked differences with such changes. This suggests that the retina by itself cannot mediate the color-spatial interactions. Although no one had seriously claimed that it could, the question continued to be debated, and it was satisfying to have some experimental evidence. The experimental results are consistent with our failure to find retinal ganglion cells that could plausibly be involved in color-spatial interactions.

The goldfish, which makes spatial comparisons very much like ours, has virtually no cerebral cortex. Perhaps the fish, unlike us, does make such computations with its retina. Nigel Daws' discovery in 1968 of *double opponent cells* in the fish retina seems to bear this out. In the monkey, as I describe in the next section, we find such cells in the cortex but not in the lateral geniculate or the retina.

BLOBS

By about 1978, the monkey's primary visual cortex, with its simple, complex, and end-stopped cells and its ocular-dominance columns and orientation columns, seemed reasonably well understood. But an unexpected feature of the physiology was that so few of the cells seemed to be interested in color. If we mapped a simple or complex cell's receptive field using white light and then repeated the mapping with colored spots or slits, the results as a rule were the same. A few cells, perhaps as many as a 10 percent of cortical upper-layer cells, did show unmistakable color preferences—with excellent responses to oriented slits of some color, most often red, and virtually no response to other wavelengths or even to white light. The orientation selectivity of these cells was just as high as that of cells lacking color selectivity. But most cells in the visual cortex did not care about color. This was all the more surprising because such a high proportion of cells in the lateral geniculate body are color coded, and the geniculate forms the main input to the visual cortex. It was hard to see what could have happened to this color information in the cortex.

Suddenly, in 1978, all this changed. Margaret Wong-Riley, at the University of California in San Francisco, discovered that when she stained the cortex for the enzyme cytochrome oxidase, the upper layers showed an unheard of inhomogeneity, with periodic dark-staining regions, pufflike in transverse cross section, about one-quarter millimeter wide and one-half millimeter apart. All cells contain cytochrome oxidase, an enzyme involved in metabolism, and no one had ever imagined that a stain for such an enzyme would show anything interesting in the cortex. When Wong-Riley sent us pictures, Torsten Wiesel and I suspected that we were seeing ocular-dominance slabs cut

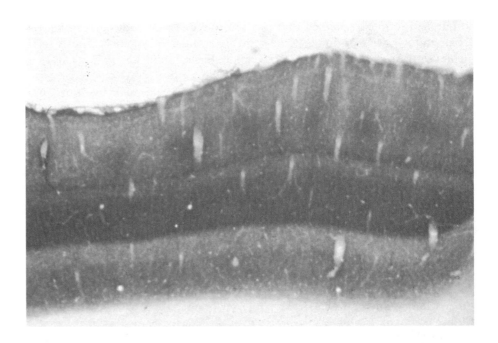

This cross section through the striate cortex shows the layers stained for the enzyme cytochrome oxidase. The darker zones in the upper third of the section are the blobs.

in cross section and that the most monocular cells were for some reason metabolically more active than binocular cells. We put the pictures in a drawer and tried to forget them.

Several years elapsed before it occurred to us or anyone else to examine the primary visual cortex with this stain in sections cut parallel to the surface. When that was finally done, roughly simultaneously by two groups (Anita Hendrickson and Alan Humphrey in Seattle and Jonathan Horton and myself in Boston), a polka-dot pattern appeared—to everyone's complete surprise. An example is shown in the photograph on this page. Instead of stripes, we saw an array of bloblike structures for which no known correlates existed. Wong-Riley's inhomogeneities have been called by almost every imaginable name: dots, puffs, patches, and spots. We call them "blobs" because the word is graphic, legitimate (appearing even in the Oxford English Dictionary), and seems to annoy our competitors.

The next task was obvious: we had to record from the striate cortex again, monitoring the experiments histologically with the cytochrome-oxidase stain to see if we could find anything different about the cells in the blobs. Margaret Livingstone and I set out to do this in 1981. The result was quite unexpected. In traversing a distance of one-quarter millimeter, the diameter of a blob, it is

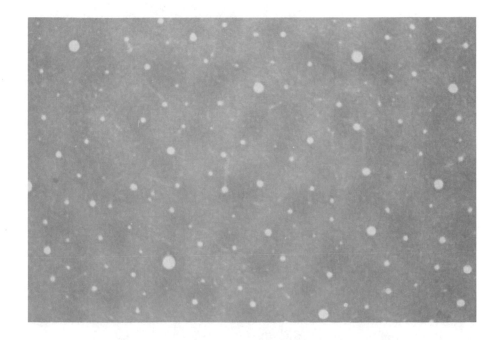

The dark areas are blobs seen face on, about 50 of which form a polka-dot pattern. This section, through layer 3 of area 17, is parallel to the cortical surface and about 0.5 millimeter beneath it. (The yellow circles are blood vessels cut transversely.)

possible to record from roughly five or six cells. Each time we crossed a blob, the cells we saw completely lacked orientation selectivity, in marked contrast to the high orientation selectivity shown by the cells outside the blobs.

One might explain this absence of orientation selectivity in either of two ways. First, these cells might receive their input unselectively from oriented cells in the nonblob neighborhood and consequently still respond specifically to lines (slits and so forth)—but by pooling all the various orientations, still end up with no preference. Second, they could resemble geniculate cells or cells in layer 4C and thus be simpler than the nonblob orientation-selective cells. The question was quickly settled: the cells were mostly center-surround. A few more experiments were enough to convince us that many of them were color coded.

Over half the blob cells had opponent-color, center-surround receptive fields, but they behaved in a decidedly more complicated way than type 1 cells in the lateral geniculate body. They gave virtually no responses to white spots of any size or shape. But to small colored spots shone in the center of the receptive field they responded vigorously over one range of wavelengths and were suppressed over another range: some were activated by long wavelengths (reds) and suppressed by short (greens and blues): others behaved in the reverse way. As with geniculate cells, we could distinguish two classes, red-green and blue-yellow, according to the position of the maximum responses. (Here, as before, red, green, and blue stand for the respective cone types, and yellow implies an input from the red and green in parallel.) So far, then, these cells closely resembled opponent-color, center-only geniculate cells (type 2). Their field centers, like centers of type 2 cells, were large—several times the size of type 1 cell centers. They were unresponsive to small shone anywhere in their receptive fields. Most surprising was the finding that these color-coded blob cells, unlike type 2 cells, were mostly unresponsive to large colored spots, regardless of wavelength content. They behaved as though each center system was surrounded by a ring of opponency. To take the commonest type, the r^+g^- center seemed to be surrounded by a ring that was r^-g^+.

Margaret Livingstone and I have called these cells *double-opponent* because of the red-green or yellow-blue opponency in the center and the antagonism of the surround to any center response, whether "on" or "off". They are therefore unresponsive not only to white light in any geometric form but also to large spots, regardless of wavelength content. As already mentioned, Nigel Daw coined the term *double-opponent* for cells he saw in the retina of the goldfish. Daw suggested that cells like these might be involved in color-spatial interactions in man, and a few years later, with Alan Pearlman, he searched carefully in the macaque monkey lateral geniculate for such cells, without success.

From the late 1960s on, double-opponent cells had occasionally been observed in the monkey cortex, but they were not clearly associated with any anatomical structure. We still do not understand some things about these cells. For example, in the r^+g^- just described, a red spot surrounded by green often gives a poor response, not the vigorous one we might expect.

Mixed with the two classes of double-opponent cells (red-green and yellow-blue) were ordinary broad-band, center-surround cells. Again, these broad-band cells differed from cells in the upper geniculate layers and from cells in $4C\beta$ in having several times larger center sizes. Blobs also contain cells that are indistinguishable from geniculate type 2 cells, resembling double-opponent cells but lacking the receptive-field surround.

Margaret Livingstone and I have proposed that the blobs represent a branch of the visual pathway that is devoted to "color", using the word broadly to include blacks, whites, and grays. This system seems to separate off from the rest of the visual path either in the lateral geniculate body or in layer 4 of the striate cortex. (The geniculate probably projects directly but weakly to the blobs. It seems likely that layer $4C\beta$ also projects to them, and it may well form their main input. Whether $4C\alpha$ projects to them is not clear.) Most blob cells seem to require border contrast in order to give responses at all: either luminous-intensity borders, in the case of the broad-band, center-surround cells or color-contrast borders, in the case of the double-opponent cells would respond. As I argued earlier, this amounts to saying that these cells play a part in color constancy.

If blob cells are involved in color constancy, they cannot be carrying out the computation exactly as Land first envisioned it, by making a separate comparison between a region and its surround for each of the cone wavebands. Instead they would seem to be doing a Hering-like comparison: of red-greenness in one region with red-greenness in the surround, and the same for yellow-blueness and for intensity. But the two ways of handling color—r, g, and b on the one hand and b-w, r-g, and y-b on the other—are really equivalent. Color requires our specifying three variables; to any color there corresponds a triplet of numbers, and we can think of any color as occupying a point in three-dimensional space. We can plot points in such a space in more than one way. The coordinate system can be Cartesian, with the three axes orthogonal and oriented in any direction or we can use polar or cylindrical coordinates. The Hering theory (and apparently the retina and brain) simply employ a different set of axes to plot the same space. This is doubtless an oversimplification because the blob cells making up the three classes are not like peas in pods but vary among themselves in the relative strengths of surrounds and centers, in their perfections in the balance between opponent colors, and in other characteristics, some still not understood. At the moment, we can only say that the physiology has a striking affinity with the psychophysics.

You may ask why the brain should go to the trouble to plot color with these seemingly weird axes rather than with the more straightforward r, g, and b axes, the way the receptor layer of the retina does. Presumably, color vision

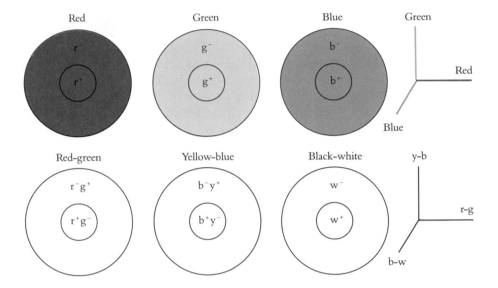

Top: Land's original formulation of the color-constancy problem seems to call for three kinds of cells, which compare the activation of a given set of cones (red, green, or blue) in one region of retina with the average activation of the same set in the surround. The result is three numbers, which specify the color at the region. Thus yellow, brown, dark gray, and olive green each has a corresponding triplet of numbers. We can therefore plot colors in a color space specified by three axes, for red, green, and blue. *Bottom:* A mathematically equivalent system also gives three numbers, and is probably closer to the way the brain specifies color. At any point on the retina, we can speak of red-greenness, the reading an instrument would give if it were to record the relative stimulation of red and green cones (zero for yellow or white). This value is determined for a particular region, and an average value is determined for the surround; then the ratio is taken. The process is repeated for yellow-blueness and black-whiteness. These three figures together are enough to specify any color.

was added in evolution to the colorless vision characteristic of lower mammals. For such animals, color space was one-dimensional, with all cone types (if the animal had more than one) pooled. When color vision evolved, two more axes were added to the one already present. It would make more sense to do that than to throw out the pooled system already present for black-white and then have to erect three new ones. When we adapt to the dark and are using only our rods, our vision becomes colorless and is again plotted along one axis, to which the rods evidently contribute. That would not be easy to do with r, g, and b axes.

At present we can only guess how double-opponent cells are wired up. For several reasons we suspect that they receive their inputs from type 2 cells: their field centers are about the same size as type 2 field centers and much larger than centers of type 1 cells; they are intermixed with type 2 cells in the blobs; and finally, as already pointed out, type 1 cells, with their opponent-color antagonistic surrounds, seem especially inappropriate as building-blocks for double-opponent receptive fields. For a red-on center double-opponent cell, the simplest arrangement, as illustrated on the facing page, would be to have excitation from one or a few red-on green-off type 2 cells whose field centers were contained within the double-opponent cell's center, and excitatory inputs from red-off green-on type 2 cells whose centers were scattered throughout the double-opponent cell's periphery. Or the surround could be formed by inhibitory inputs from red-on green-off type 2 cells. (Originally we favored a scheme in which the inputs were made up of type 1 cells. Logically such an arrangement is possible, but it seems much more awkward.)

This leaves unsettled the part that type 1 cells play in color vision—if they play any part at all. These are the most common cells in the lateral geniculate body, and they supply the lion's share of the input to the visual cortex. Their obvious color coding makes it easy to lose sight of the fact that they are beautifully organized to respond to light-dark contours, which they do with great precision. Indeed, in the fovea, where their centers are fed by one cone only, they have no choice but to be color-coded. (The mystery is why the surround should be supplied by a single, different, cone type; it would seem more reasonable for the surrounds to be broad-band.) Given this massively color-coded input it is astonishing that interblob cells in the cortex show so little interest in color. The few exceptions respond to red slits but not to white ones, and are thus clearly color coded. For the most part it would seem that the information on wavelength carried by type 1 cells is pooled, and the information about color lost. In one sense, however, it is not discarded completely. In Freiburg, in 1979, Jürgen Krüger and Peter Gouras showed that cortical cells often respond to lines formed by appropriately oriented red-green (or orange-green) borders at all relative intensities of red and green. A truly color blind cell, like a color blind person, should be insensitive to the border at the ratio of intensities to which the cones respond equally. These cells presumably use the type 1 color information to allow contours of equal luminance to be visible by virtue of wavelength differences alone—of obvious value in defeating attempts at camouflage by predators or prey.

The recognition of colors as such would thus seem to be an ability distinct from the ability to detect color borders, and to require a separate pathway consisting of type 2 cells and color-opponent blob cells. Our tendency to think of color and form as separate aspects of perception thus has its counterpart in the physical segregation of blobs and nonblob regions in the primary visual cortex. Beyond the striate cortex the segregation is perpetuated, in visual area 2 and even beyond that. We do not know where, or if, they combine.

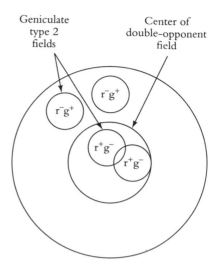

Geniculate type 2 fields

Center of double-opponent field

A double-opponent cell could be built up from many geniculate type 2 cells. If the cell is r^+g^- center, r^-g^+ surround, then its inputs could be a large number of r^+g^- type 2 cells with fields scattered throughout the cell's receptive field center, and r^-g^+ type 2 cells with fields scattered throughout the cell's receptive field surround, all making excitatory contacts with the double-opponent cell. Alternatively, the surround could be formed from r^+g^- type 2 cells, making inhibitory contacts.

CONCLUSION

The subject of color vision illustrates so well the possibilities of understanding otherwise quite mysterious phenomena—the results of color mixing or the constancy of colors despite changes in the light source—by using a combination of psychophysical and neurophysiological methods. For all their complexity, the problems presented by color are probably simpler than those presented by form. Despite all the orientation-specific and end-stopped cells, we are still a long way from understanding our ability to recognize shapes, to distinguish shapes from their background, or to interpret three dimensions from the flat pictures presented to each of our eyes. To compare the modalities of color and form at all may itself be misleading: remember that differences in color at borders without any differences in luminous intensity, can lead to perception of shapes. Thus color, like black and white, is just one means by which shapes manifest themselves.

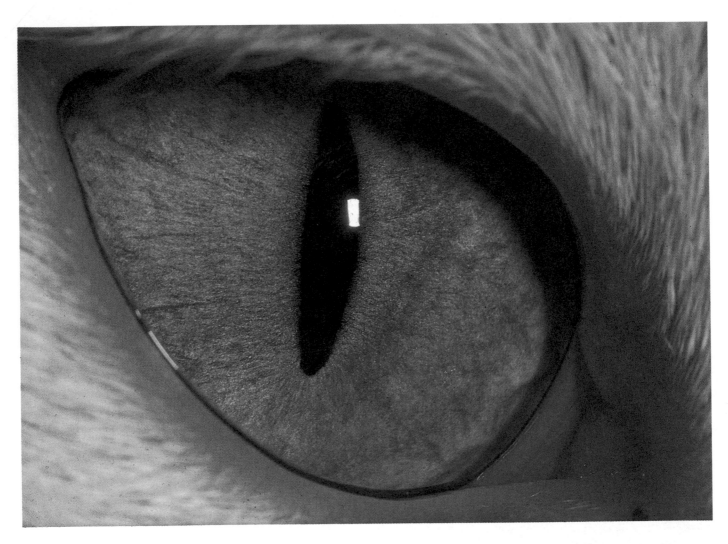

The slit shape of the pupil found in many nocturnal animals such as this cat presumably allows more effective light reduction than a circular pupil.

9

DEPRIVATION AND DEVELOPMENT

Up to now we have been thinking of the brain as a fully formed, mature machine. We have been asking how it is connected, how the parts function in terms of everyday situations, and how they serve the interests of the animal. But that leaves untouched an entirely different and most important question: How did the machine get there in the first place?

The problem has two major components. Much of the brain's development has to go on in the mother's uterus, before the animal is born. A glance at the brain of a newborn human tells us that although it has fewer creases and is somewhat smaller than the adult brain, it is otherwise not very different. But a glance can hardly tell us the whole story, because the baby is certainly not born knowing the alphabet or able to play tennis or the harp. All these accomplishments take training, and by training, we surely mean the molding or modification of neuronal circuits by environmental influences. The ultimate form of the brain, then, is a result of both prenatal and postnatal development. First, it involves a maturation that takes care of itself, depends on intrinsic properties of the organism, and occurs before or after the time at which birth happens to occur; second, it involves postnatal maturation that depends on instruction, training, education, learning, and experience—all more or less synonymous terms.

Prenatal development is a gargantuan subject; I know little about it and certainly will not attempt to describe it in any detail here. One of the more interesting but baffling topics it deals with is the question of how the individual nerve fibers in a huge bundle find their proper destinations. For example, the eye, the geniculate, and the cortex are all formed independently of each other: as one of them matures, the axons that grow out must make many decisions. An optic-nerve fiber must grow across the retina to the optic disc, then along the optic nerve to the chiasm, deciding there whether to cross or not; it must then proceed to the lateral geniculate body on the side it has selected, go to the right layer or to the region that will become the right layer, go to just the right part of that layer so that the resulting topography becomes properly ordered, and finally it must branch and the branches must go to the correct parts of the geniculate cells—cell body or dendrite. The same requirements apply to a fiber growing from the lateral geniculate body to area 17 or from area 17 to area 18. Although this general aspect of neurodevelopment is today receiving intense study in many laboratories, we still do not know how fibers seek out their targets. It is hard even to guess the winner out of the several major possibilities, mechanical guidance, following chemical gradients, or homing in on some complementary molecule in a manner analogous to what happens in immune systems. Much present-day research seems to point to many mechanisms, not just to one.

This chapter deals mainly with the postnatal development of the mammalian visual system, in particular with the degree to which the system can be affected by the environment. In the first few stages of the cat and monkey visual path—the retina, geniculate, and perhaps the striate, or primary visual, cortex—an obvious question is whether any plasticity should be expected after birth. I will begin by describing a simple experiment. By about 1962 some of the main facts about the visual cortex of the adult cat were known: orientation selectivity had been discovered, simple and complex cells had been distinguished, and many cortical cells were known to be binocular and to show varying degrees of eye preference. We knew enough about the adult animal that we could ask direct questions aimed at learning whether the visual system was malleable. So Torsten Wiesel and I took a kitten a week old, when the eyes were just about to open, and sewed shut the lids of one eye. The procedure sounds harsh, but it was done under anesthesia and the kitten showed no signs of discomfort or distress when it woke up, back with its mother and littermates. After ten weeks we reopened the eye surgically, again under an anesthetic, and recorded from the kitten's cortex to learn whether the eye closure had had any effect on the eye or on the visual path.

Before I describe the results, I should explain that a long history of research in psychology and of observations in clinical neurology prompted this experiment. Psychologists had experimented extensively with visual deprivation in animals in the 1940s and 1950s, using behavioral methods to assess the effects. A typical experiment was to bring animals up from birth in complete darkness. When the animals were brought out into the light, they turned out to be blind or at least very defective visually. The blindness was to some extent reversible, but only slowly and not in most cases completely.

Paralleling these experiments were clinical observations on children born with cataracts. A cataract is a condition in which the lens of the eye becomes milky, transmitting light but no longer permitting an image to form on the retina. Cataracts in newborns, like those in adults, are treated by removing the lenses surgically and compensating by fitting the child with an artificial lens implant or with thick glasses. In that way, a perfectly focused retinal image can be restored. Although the operation is relatively easy, ophthalmologists have been loath to do it in very young infants or babies, mainly because any operation at a very early age carries more risk statistically, although the risk is small. When cataracts were removed, say at an age of eight years, and glasses fitted, the results were bitterly disappointing. Eyesight was not restored at all: the child was blind as ever, and profound deficits persisted even after months or years of attempts to learn to see. A child would, for example, continue to be unable to tell a circle from a triangle. With hopes thus raised and dashed, the child was generally worse off, not better. We can contrast this with clinical experience in adults: a man of seventy-five develops cataracts and gradually loses sight in both eyes. After three years of blindness the cataracts are removed, glasses fitted, and vision is completely restored. The vision can even be better than it was before the cataracts developed, because all lenses yellow with age, and their removal results in a sky of marvelous blue seen otherwise only by children and young adults.

It would seem that visual deprivation in children has adverse effects of a sort that do not occur at all in adults. Psychologists commonly and quite reasonably attributed the results of their experiments, as well as the clinical results, to a failure of the child to learn to see or, presumably the equivalent, to a failure of connections to develop for want of some kind of training experience.

Amblyopia is a partial or complete loss of eyesight that is not caused by abnormalities in the eye. When we sewed closed a cat's or monkey's eye, our aim was to produce an amblyopia and then to try to learn where the abnormality had arisen in the visual path. The results of the kitten experiment amazed us. All too often, an experiment gives wishy-washy results, too good to dismiss completely but too indecisive to let us conclude anything useful. This experiment was an exception; the results were clear and dramatic. When we opened the lids of the kitten's eye, the eye itself seemed perfectly normal: the pupil even contracted normally when we shined a light into it. Recordings from the cortex, however, were anything but normal. Although we found many cells with perfectly normal responses to oriented lines and movement, we also found that instead of about half of the cells preferring one eye and half preferring the other, none of the twenty-five cells we recorded could be influenced from the eye that had been closed. (Five of the cells could not be influenced from either eye, something that we see rarely if ever in normal cats.) Compare this with a normal cat, in which about 15 percent of cells are monocular, with about 7 percent responding to the left eye and 7 percent to the right. The ocular-dominance histograms for the cat, shown in the top graph on the

A kitten (top histograms) was visually deprived after having its right eye closed at
about ten days, the time at which the eyes
normally open. The duration of closure
was two-and-a-half months. In this experiment we recorded from only twenty-five
cells. (In subsequent experiments we were
able to record more cells, and we found a
small percentage that were influenced from
the eye that had been closed.) The results
were very similar for a baby monkey (bottom histograms). It had its right eye closed
at two weeks, and the eye remained closed
for eighteen months. We subsequently
found that the result is the same if the eye
is closed for only a few weeks.

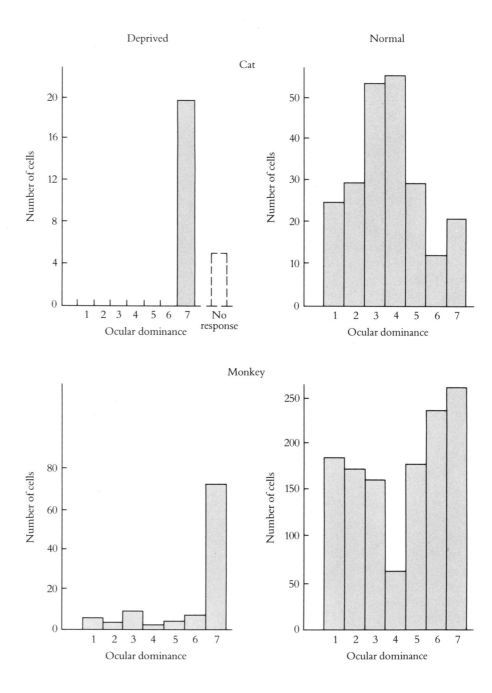

facing page, allowed us to see the difference at a glance. Clearly something had gone wrong, with a vengeance.

We soon repeated the experiment in more kittens and in baby monkeys. In kittens, a larger series soon showed that if an eye is closed at birth, on the average only 15 percent of cells prefer the eye that was closed, instead of about 50 percent. The same results were found in monkeys (see the bottom histogram). Of the few cells that did respond through the eye that had been closed, many seemed abnormal; they fired sluggishly, fatigued easily, and lacked the normal precise orientation tuning.

A result like this raises many questions. Where in the visual path was the abnormality? In the eye? The cortex? Could the cat see with the eye that had been closed, despite the cortical abnormality? Was it light or form deprivation that produced the abnormality? Was the age at which we closed the eye important? Was the abnormality a result of disuse or of something else? To get answers to such questions took a long time, but we can state the results in a few words.

The obvious way to determine the site of the abnormality was to record at lower levels, starting, say, in the eye or the geniculate. The results were unequivocal: both the eye and the geniculate had plenty of cells whose responses were virtually normal. Cells in the geniculate layers that received input from the eye that had been closed had the usual center-surround receptive fields; they responded well to a small spot and poorly to diffuse light. The only hint of abnormality was a slight sluggishness in the responses of these cells, compared with the responses of cells in the layers fed by the normal eye.

Given this relative normality, we were amazed when we first saw the Nissl-stained lateral geniculate under the microscope. It was so abnormal that a microscope was hardly needed. The cat's geniculate has a somewhat more simple organization than the monkey's; it consists mainly of two large-cell layers, which are on top rather than on the bottom, as in the monkey. The upper layer receives input from the contralateral eye, the lower from the ipsilateral. Beneath these layers is a rather poorly defined small-cell layer with several subdivisions, which I will ignore here. On each side, the large-cell layer receiving input from the closed eye was pale and clearly thinner than its companion, which looked robust and perfectly normal. The cells in the abnormal layers were not only pale but were shriveled to about two-thirds their normal cross-sectional area. This result for a right-eye closure is shown in the photographs on the next page. Similar results were found in the macaque monkey for a right-eye closure, as shown in the photograph on page 197. We thus faced a paradox that took us a few years to explain: a lateral geniculate whose cells seemed relatively normal physiologically but were manifestly pathological histologically. Our original question was in any case answered, since cortical cells, although virtually unresponsive to the closed eye, were evidently receiv-

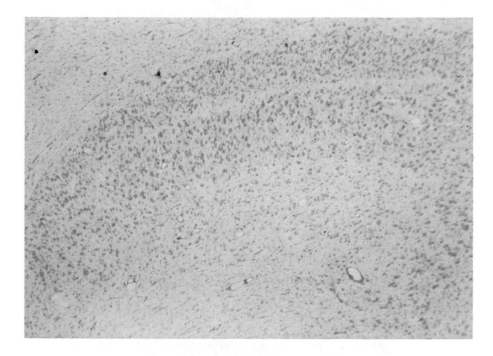

The lateral geniculate bodies of a kitten show obvious abnormalities when the right eye has been closed at ten days for three-and-a-half months. The two main layers can be seen in the top half of the photographs. *Top:* In the left geniculate the upper layer (contralateral to the closed, right eye) is shrivelled and pale staining. *Bottom:* In the right geniculate the lower of the two layers (ipsilateral) is abnormal. The two layers together are about 1 millimeter thick. The ocular-dominance histogram is shown on page 194.

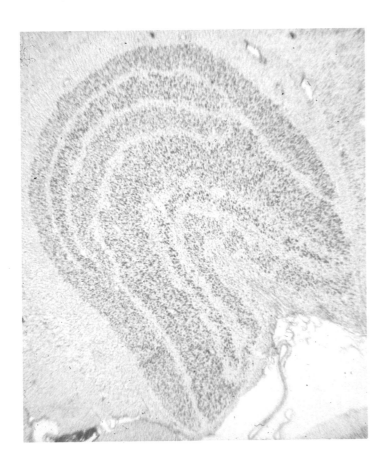 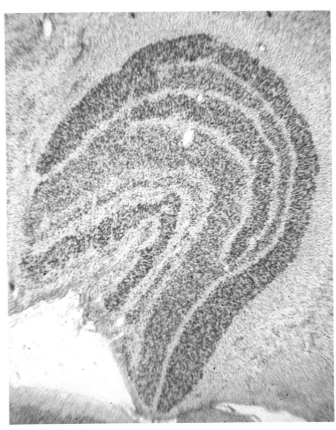

ing a substantial and, on the face of it, practically normal geniculate input. This seemed to exonerate both the eye and the geniculate as primary sites of the damage and placed the main abnormality in the cortex. When we looked at the cortex histologically, we saw absolutely nothing to suggest any abnormality. As we will see, the cortex does show anatomical defects, but they do not show up with these staining methods.

We next asked what it was about the eye closures that produced the abnormality. Closing the eye reduces the light reaching the retina by a factor of about ten to fifty; of course, it also prevents any images from reaching the retina. Could it be simply the reduction in light that was causing the trouble? To help decide, we inserted in one eye of a newborn kitten an opalescent contact lens made of a plastic with the consistency of a ping pong ball. In some animals we instead surgically sewed over one eye a thin, translucent, opalescent membrane, in effect, an extra eyelid called the nictitating membrane that

Abnormal layers appear in the left and right lateral geniculate bodies (seen in cross section) of a monkey whose right eye was closed at age two weeks for eighteen months. On both sides, the layers receiving input from the eye that was closed (the right eye) are paler: layers 1, 4, and 6 on the left; layers 2, 3, and 5 on the right, numbered from below. The cells in the affected layers are smaller, but this cannot be seen at such low power. The width of the entire structure is about 5 millimeters.

cats possess and we don't. The plastic or the membrane reduced the light by about one-half but prevented the formation of any focused images. The results were the same: an abnormal cortical physiology; an abnormal geniculate histology. Evidently it was the form deprivation rather than light deprivation that was doing the damage.

In a few kittens we tested vision before recording by putting an opaque black contact lens over the eye that had not been closed and then observing how the animal made out. The animals were clearly blind in the eye that had been deprived: they would walk confidently over to the edge of a low table, go past the edge, and fall to a mattress placed on the floor. On the floor they would walk into table legs. These are things no normal, self-respecting cat ever does. Similar tests with the eye that had not been closed showed that vision was entirely normal.

Next we did a protracted study in both cats and monkeys to learn whether the age at which the closures were done and the duration of the closures were important. It soon became clear that age of onset of deprivation was critical. An adult cat deprived of vision in one eye for over a year developed no blindness in that eye, no loss of responses in the cortex, and no geniculate pathology. (The first cat we deprived, the mother of our first litter of kittens, was an adult by definition.) We concluded after many experiments that somewhere between birth and adulthood there must be a period of plasticity during which deprivation produces the cortical deficit. For the cat, this *critical period* turned out to be between the fourth week and the fourth month. Not surprisingly, closing an eye had little effect prior to the fourth week, because a cat uses its vision hardly at all during the first month of its life: the eyes open only around the tenth day, and for the next few weeks the kittens are behind the sofa with their mother. The susceptibility to deprivation comes on quickly and reaches a maximum in the first few weeks of the critical period. During that time, even a few days of closure result in a palpably distorted ocular-dominance histogram. Over the ensuing four months or so, the duration of closure required to give obvious effects increases steadily; in other words, the susceptibility to deprivation tapers off.

The histograms summarizing some of the results in monkeys can be seen in the three graphs on the facing page. The left graph shows the severe effects of a six-week closure done at five days; almost no cells could be driven from the eye that was closed. A much briefer early closure (middle graph) also gave severe effects, but clearly not quite as severe as the longer closure. At four months the susceptibility begins to wane, so much so that even a closure of five years' duration, as shown in the righthand graph, although giving pronounced effects, is no match for the results of the earlier closure.

In these studies of the time course of the sensitive period, cats and monkeys gave very similar results. In the monkey, the sensitive period began earlier, at

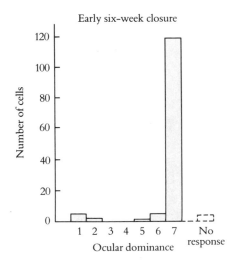

Early six-week closure

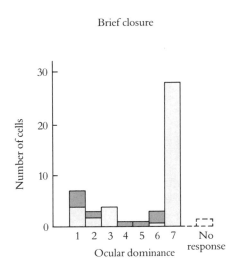

Brief closure

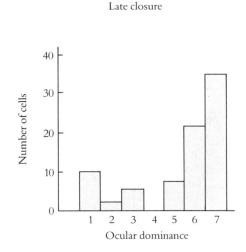

Late closure

Left: The left eye is almost completely dominant in a monkey whose right eye was sutured closed at an age of five days, for six weeks. *Middle:* A closure of only a few days in a monkey a few weeks old is enough to produce a marked shift in ocular dominance. Darker shading indicates the number of abnormal cells. *Right:* If the closure of the monkey's eye is delayed until age four months, even a very long closure (in this case five years) results in an eye-dominance shift that is far less marked than that resulting from a brief closure at an age of a few weeks.

birth rather than at four weeks, and lasted longer, gradually tapering off over the first year instead of at around four months. It reached its peak in the first two weeks of life, during which even a few days of closure was enough to give a marked shift in ocular dominance. Closing the eye of an adult monkey produced no ill effects, regardless of the duration of closure. In one adult monkey, we closed an eye for four years, with no blindness, cortical deficit, or geniculate-cell shrinkage.

RECOVERY

We next asked whether any recovery in physiology in a monkey could be obtained by opening the eye that had been closed. The answer was that after a week or more of eye closure, little or no physiological recovery ever occurred if the closed eye was simply opened and nothing else done. Even a few years later, the cortex was about as abnormal as it would have been at the time of reopening the eye, as shown in the left graph on the next page. If at the time of reopening, the other, originally open eye was closed, in a procedure

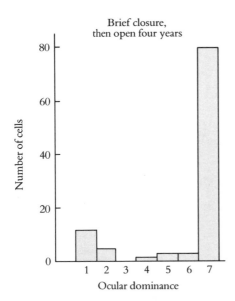

Brief closure,
then open four years

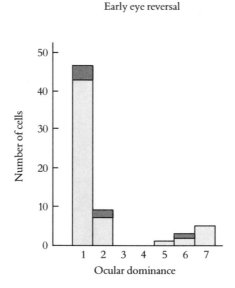

Early eye reversal

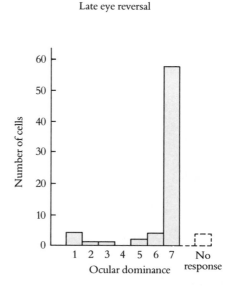

Late eye reversal

One eye was closed at birth for nine days in this monkey and then opened. The recordings were done four years later, during which time the animal had had much testing of its vision. Even that long a period with both eyes open produced little recovery in the physiology.

The right eye in this macaque monkey was closed at birth. At five and a half weeks the right eyelids were opened and the left closed. When at six months the recording was made from the right hemisphere, most of the cells strongly favored the right, originally closed eye.

In this macaque monkey the right eye was closed at seven days, for one year, at which time the right eye was opened and the left was closed. After another year, the left eye was opened, and both remained open. When finally the recording was made at three and a half years, most cells favored the eye that was originally open. Evidently one year is too late to do a reverse suture.

called *eye reversal,* recovery did occur but only if the reversal was done when the monkey was still in the critical period, as shown in the middle and right-hand graphs above for early and late eye reversal. After the critical period, even an eye reversal followed by several years with the second eye closed failed to bring about anything more than slight recovery in the anatomy or physiology.

The monkey's ability to see did not necessarily closely parallel the cortical physiology. Without reversal, the originally closed eye never recovered its sight. With reversal, sight did return and often approached normal levels, but this was so even in late reversals, in which the physiology remained very abnormal in the originally closed eye. We still do not understand this disparity between the lack of substantial physiological or anatomical recovery and what in some cases seemed to be considerable restoration of vision. Perhaps the two sets of tests are measuring different things. We tested the acuity of vision by measuring the ability to discriminate such things as the smallest detectable gap in a line or circle. But testing this type of acuity may yield an incomplete measure of visual function. It seems hard to believe that such florid physiological and anatomical deficits in function and structure would be reflected behaviorally by nothing more than the minor fall in acuity we measured.

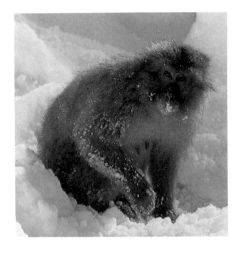

The Japanese macaque monkey, *Macaca fuscata,* the largest of all macaques, lives on the ground and in trees in northern Japan. It is protected by its thick grey-brown coat.

THE NATURE OF THE DEFECT

The results I have been describing made it clear that a lack of images on the retina early in life led to profound long-lasting defects in cortical function. These results nevertheless left open two major questions concerning the nature of the underlying process. The first of these was a "nature versus nurture" question: Were we depriving our animals of an experience that they needed in order to build the right connections, or were we destroying or disrupting connections that were already present, prewired and functional at the time the animal was born? The dark-rearing experiments done in the decades prior to our work had practically all been interpreted in the context of learning—or failure to learn. The cerebral cortex, where most people thought (and still think) that memory and mental activity resides, was looked upon in roughly the same way as the 1-megabyte memory board for which we pay so much when we buy our computers: these contain many elements and connections, but no information, until we put it there. In short, people regarded the cortex as a *tabula rasa.*

One obvious way to decide between these alternatives is to address the question head on and simply record from a newborn cat or monkey. If learning is necessary for the wiring up to occur, then we should fail to find any of the rich specificity that we see in adult animals. A lack of specificity would nevertheless not decide the issue, because we could then ascribe the lack of connections either to immaturity—still-incomplete genetically programmed wiring—or to lack of experience. On the other hand, finding such specificity would argue against a learning mechanism. We did not expect the experiments with kittens to be easy, and they weren't. Kittens are visually very immature at birth and make no use at all of their eyes before about the tenth day, when the eyes open. At that time, even the media of the eye, the transparent substances between the cornea and the retina, are far from clear, so that it is impossible to get a clear image on the retina. The immature visual cortex indeed responded sluggishly and somewhat unpredictably and was on the whole a far cry from a normal adult visual cortex; nevertheless we found many clearly orientation-specific cells. The more days that elapsed between birth and recording, the

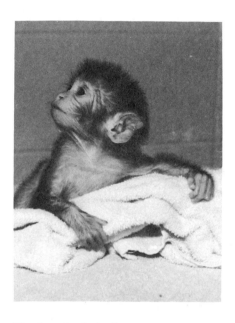

The day after its birth, a macaque monkey is looking about, fixating on objects, taking a keen interest in his environment. Humans and cats show this degree of visual maturity only many weeks after birth.

more the cells behaved like adult cells: perhaps because the media were clearer and the animal more robust but perhaps because learning had occurred. Interpretations differed from one set of observers to another.

The most convincing evidence came from newborn monkeys. The day after it is born, a macaque monkey is visually remarkably mature: unlike a newborn cat or human, it looks, follows objects, and takes a keen interest in its surroundings. Consistent with this behavior, the cells in the neonate monkey's primary visual cortex seemed about as sharply orientation-tuned as in the adult. The cells even showed precise, orderly sequences of orientation shifts (see the graph on this page). We did see differences between newborn and adult animals, but the system of receptive-field orientation, the hallmark of striate cortical function, seemed to be well organized.

Compared with that of the newborn cat or human, the newborn macaque monkey's visual system may be mature, but it certainly differs anatomically from the visual system of the adult monkey. A Nissl-stained section of cortex looks different: the layers are thinner and the cells packed closer. As Simon LeVay first observed, even the total area of the striate cortex expands by about 30 percent between birth and adulthood. If we stain the cortex by the Golgi method or examine it under an electron microscope, the differences are even more obvious: cells typically have a sparser dendritic tree and fewer synapses. Given these differences, we would be surprised if the cortex at birth behaved exactly as it does in an adult. On the other hand, dendrites and synapses are still sparser and fewer a month before birth. The nature-nurture question is whether postnatal development depends on experience or goes on even after birth according to a built-in program. We still are not sure of the answer, but from the relative normality of responses at birth, we can conclude that the unresponsiveness of cortical cells after deprivation was mainly due to a deteri-

In a newborn macaque monkey, the cortical cells seem about as sharply tuned for orientation as in adult monkeys, and the sequences are about as orderly.

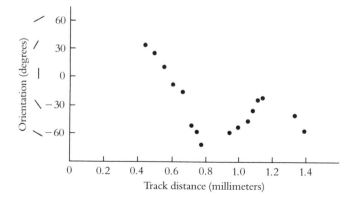

oration of connections that had been present at birth, not to a failure to form because of lack of experience.

The second major question had to do with the cause of this deterioration. At first glance, the answer seemed almost obvious. We supposed that the deterioration came about through disuse, just as leg muscles atrophy if the knee or ankle is immobilized in a cast. The geniculate-cell shrinkage was presumably closely related to *postsynaptic atrophy,* the cell shrinkage seen in the lateral geniculates of adult animals or humans after an eye is removed. It turned out that these assumptions were wrong. The assumptions had seemed so self-evident that I'm not sure we ever would have thought of designing an experiment to test them. We were forced to change our minds only because we did what seemed to us at the time an unnecessary experiment, for reasons that I forget.

We sutured closed both eyes, first in a newborn cat and later in a newborn monkey. If the cortical unresponsiveness in the path from one eye arose from disuse, sewing up both eyes should give double the defect: we should find virtually no cells that responded to the left or to the right eye. To our great surprise, the result was anything but unresponsive cells: we found a cortex in which fully half the cells responded normally, one quarter responded abnormally, and one quarter did not respond at all. We had to conclude that you cannot predict the fate of a cortical cell when an eye is closed unless you are told whether the other eye has been closed too. Close one eye, and the cell is almost certain to lose its connections from that eye; close both, and the chances are good that the control will be preserved. Evidently we were dealing not with disuse, but with some kind of eye competition. It was as if a cell began by having two sets of synaptic inputs, one from each eye, and with one pathway not used, the other took over, preempting the territory of the first pathway, as shown in the drawing on this page.

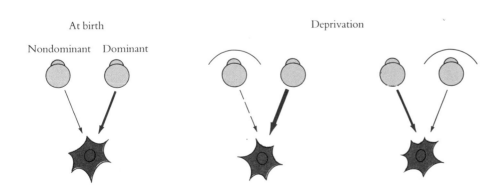

At birth

Nondominant Dominant

Deprivation

We suppose a cortical cell receives input from two sources, one from each eye, and that covering one eye has the effect of weakening the connections from that eye and strengthening the connections from the other one.

Such reasoning, we thought, could hardly apply to the geniculate shrinkage because geniculate cells are monocular, with no obvious opportunities for competition. For the time being we could not explain the cell shrinkage in the layers corresponding to the closed eye. With binocular closure, the shrinkage of geniculate cells seemed less conspicuous, but it was hard to be sure because we had no normal layers to use as a standard of comparison. Our understanding of this whole problem did not move ahead until we began to use some of the new methods of experimental anatomy.

STRABISMUS

The commonest cause of amblyopia in humans is *strabismus,* or *squint,* terms that signify nonparallel eyes—cross-eye or wall-eye. (The term *squint* as technically used is synonymous with strabismus and has nothing to do with squinching up the eyes in bright light.) The cause of strabismus is unknown, and indeed it probably has more than one cause. In some cases, strabismus comes on shortly after birth, during the first few months when in humans the eyes would just be starting to fixate and follow objects. The lack of straightness could be the result of an abnormality in the eye muscles, or it could be caused by a derangement in the circuits in the brainstem that subserve eye movements.

In some children, strabismus seems to be the result of long-sightedness. To focus properly at a distance, the lens in a long-sighted eye has to become as globular as the lens of a normal eye becomes when it focuses on a near object. To round up the lens for close work means contracting the ciliary muscle inside the eye, which is called *accommodation.* When a normal person accommodates to focus on something close, the eyes automatically also turn in, or *converge.* The figure on the facing page shows the two processes. The circuits in the brainstem for accommodation and convergence are probably related and may overlap; in any case, it is hard to do one without doing the other. When a long-sighted person accommodates, as he must to focus even on a distant object, one or both eyes may turn in, even though the convergence in this case is counterproductive. If a long-sighted child is not fitted with glasses, turning in an eye may become habitual and eventually permanent. This explanation for strabismus must surely be valid for some cases, but not for all, since strabismus is not necessarily accompanied by long-sightedness and since in some people with strabismus, one or other eye turns out rather than in.

Strabismus can be treated surgically by detaching and reattaching the extraocular muscles. The operation is usually successful in straightening the eyes, but until the last decade or so it was not generally done until a child had

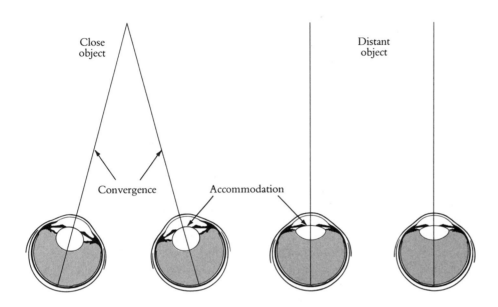

Close
object

Distant
object

Convergence   Accommodation

When we look at a near object two things happen: the lens rounds up because ciliary muscles contract, and the eyes turn in.

reached the age of four to ten, for the same reason that cataract removal was delayed—the slight increase in risk.

Strabismus that arises in an adult, say from an injury to a nerve or eye muscle, is of course accompanied by double vision. To see what that is like, you need only press (gently) on one eye from below and one side. Double vision can be most annoying and incapacitating, and if no better solution is available, a patch may have to be put over one eye, as in the Hathaway shirt man. The double vision otherwise persists as long as the strabismus is uncorrected. In a child with strabismus, however, the double vision rarely persists; instead, either alternation or suppression of vision in one eye occurs.

When a child alternates, he fixes (directs his gaze) first with one eye, while the nonfixating eye turns in or out, and then fixes with the other while the first eye is diverted. (Alternating strabismus is very common, and once you know about the condition, you can easily recognize it.) The eyes take turns fixating, perhaps every second or so, and while one eye is looking, the other seems not to see. At any instant, with one eye straight and the other deviating, vision in the deviated eye is said to be *suppressed*. Suppression is familiar to anyone who has trained himself to look through a monocular microscope, sight a gun, or do any other strictly one-eye task, with the other eye open. The scene simply disappears for the suppressed eye. A child who alternates is always suppressing one or other eye, but if we test vision separately in each eye, we generally find both eyes to be normal.

Some children with strabismus do not alternate but use one eye all the time, suppressing the other eye. When one eye is habitually suppressed, vision tends to deteriorate in the suppressed eye. Acuity falls, especially in or near the central, or foveal part of the visual field, and if the situation continues, the eye may become for practical purposes blind. This kind of blindness is what the ophthalmologists call *amblyopia ex anopsia*. It is by far the commonest kind of amblyopia, indeed of blindness in general.

It was natural for us to think of trying to induce strabismus, and hence amblyopia, in a kitten or monkey by surgically cutting an eye muscle at birth, since we could then look at the physiology and see what part of the path had failed. We did this in half a dozen kittens and were discouraged to find that the kittens, like many children, developed alternating strabismus; they looked first with one eye and then the other. By testing each eye separately, we soon verified that they had normal vision in both eyes. Evidently we had failed to induce an amblyopia, and we debated what to do next. We decided to record from one of the kittens, even though we had no idea what we could possibly learn. (Research often consists of groping.) The results were completely unexpected. As we recorded from cell after cell, we soon realized that something strange had happened to the brain: each cell responded completely normally, but only through one eye. As the electrode advanced through the cortex, cell after cell would respond from the left eye, then suddenly the sequence would be broken and the other eye would take over. Unlike what we had seen after eye closure, neither eye seemed to have suffered relative to the other eye in terms of its overall hegemony. Binocular cells occasionally appeared near the points of transition, but in the kittens, the proportion of binocular cells in the population was about 20 percent instead of the normal 85 percent, as shown in the graph on this page.

We wondered whether most of the originally binocular cells had simply died or become unresponsive, leaving behind only monocular cells. This seemed very unlikely because as the electrode advanced, the cortex of these animals yielded the usual richness of responding cells: it did not seem at all like a cortex depleted of four-fifths of its cells. In a normal cat, in a typical penetration parallel to the surface in the upper layers, we see about ten to fifteen cells in a row—all dominated by the same eye, all obviously belonging to the same ocular-dominance column—of which two or three may be monocular. In the strabismic animals we likewise saw ten to fifteen cells all dominated by one eye, but now all but two to three were monocular. Each cell had apparently come to be dominated completely or almost completely by the eye it had originally merely preferred.

To appreciate the surprising quality of this result you have to remember that we had not really interfered with the total amount of visual stimulus reaching either retina. Because we had no reason to think that we had injured either eye,

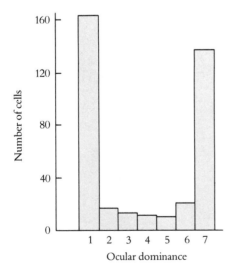

After we cut one eye muscle in a kitten at birth and then recorded after three months, the great majority of cells were monocular, falling into groups 1 and 7.

we assumed, correctly as it turned out, that the overall traffic of impulses in the two optic nerves must have been normal.

How, then, could the strabismus have produced such a radical change in cortical function? To answer this we need to consider how the two eyes normally act together. What the strabismus had changed was the relationship between the stimuli to the two eyes. When we look at a scene, the images in the two retinas from any point in the scene normally fall on locations that are the same distance and in the same direction from the two foveas—they fall on corresponding points. If a binocular cell in the cortex happens to be activated when an image falls on the left retina—if the cell's receptive field is crossed by a dark-light contour whose orientation is exactly right for the cell—then that cell will also be excited by the image on the right retina, for three reasons: (1) the images fall on the same parts of the two retinas, (2) a binocular cell (unless it is specialized for depth) has its receptive fields in exactly the same parts of the two retinas, and (3) the orientation preferences of binocular cells are always the same in the two eyes. If the eyes are not parallel, reason 1 obviously no longer applies: with the images no longer in concordance, if at a given moment a cell happens to be told to fire by one eye, whether the other eye will also be telling the cell to fire is a matter of chance. This, as far as a single cell is concerned, would seem to be the only thing that changes in strabismus. Somehow, in a young kitten, the perpetuation over weeks or months of this state of affairs, in which the signals from the two eyes are no longer concordant, causes the weaker of the two sets of connections to the cell to weaken even further and often for practical purposes to disappear. Thus we have an example of ill effects coming not as a result of removing or withholding a stimulus, but merely as a result of disrupting the normal time relationships between two sets of stimuli—a subtle insult indeed, considering the gravity of the consequences.

In these experiments, monkeys gave the same results as kittens; it therefore seems likely that strabismus leads to the same consequences in humans. Clinically, in someone with a long-standing alternating strabismus, even if the strabismus is repaired, the person does not usually regain the ability to see depth. The surgeon can bring the two eyes into alignment only to the nearest few degrees. Perhaps the failure to recover is due to the loss of the person's ability to make up the residual deficit, to fuse the two images perfectly by bringing the eyes into alignment to the nearest few minutes of arc. Surgically repairing the strabismus aligns the eyes well enough so that in a normal person the neural mechanisms would be sufficient to take care of the remaining few degrees of fine adjustment, but in a strabismic person these are the very mechanisms, including binocular cells in the cortex, that have been disrupted. To get recovery would presumably require protracted reestablishment of perfect alignment in the two eyes, something that requires normal muscle alignment plus an alignment depending on binocular vision.

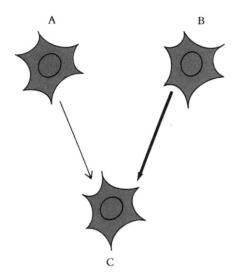

Cell C receives inputs from A, a left-eye cell, and B, a right-eye cell. The Hebb synapse model says that if cell C fires after cell A fires, the sequence of events will tend to strengthen the A-to-C synapse.

This model for explaining a cell's shift in ocular dominance is strongly reminiscent of a synaptic-level model for explaining associative learning. Known as the *Hebb synapse* model, after psychologist Donald Hebb of McGill University, its essential idea is that a synapse between two neurons, A and C, will become more effective the more often an incoming signal in nerve A is followed by an impulse in nerve C, regardless of exactly why nerve C fires (see the illustration on this page). Thus for the synapse to improve, nerve C need not fire *because* A fired. Suppose, for example, that a second nerve, B, makes a synapse with C, and the A-to-C synapse is weak and the B-to-C synapse is strong; suppose further that A and B fire at about the same time or that B fires just slightly ahead of A and that C then fires not because of the effects of A but because of the strong effects of B. In a Hebb synapse, the mere fact that C fires immediately after A makes the A-to-C synapse stronger. We also suppose that if impulses coming in via path A are not followed by impulses in C, the A-to-C synapse becomes weaker.

To apply this model to binocular convergence in the normal animal, we let cell C be binocular, nerve A be from the nondominant eye, and nerve B be from the dominant eye. The nondominant eye is less likely than the dominant eye to fire the cell. The Hebb hypothesis says that the synapse between nerves A and C will be maintained or strengthened as long as an impulse in A is followed by an impulse in C, an event that is more likely to occur if help consistently comes from the other eye, nerve B, at the right time. And that, in turn, will happen if the eyes are aligned. If activity in A is not followed by activity in C, in the long run the synapse between A and C will be weakened. It may not be easy to get direct proof that the Hebb synapse model applies to strabismus, at least not in the near future, but the idea seems attractive.

THE ANATOMICAL CONSEQUENCES OF DEPRIVATION

Our failure to find any marked physiological defects in geniculate cells, where little or no opportunity exists for eye competition, seemed to uphold the idea that the effects of monocular eye closure reflected competition rather than disuse. To be sure, the geniculate cells were histologically atrophic, but—so we rationalized—one could not expect everything to fit. If competition was indeed the important thing, it seemed that cortical layer 4C might provide a good place to test the idea, for here, too, the cells were monocular and competition was therefore unlikely, so that the alternating left-eye, right-eye stripes should be undisturbed. Thus by recording in long microelectrode tracks through layer 4C, we set out to learn whether the patches still existed after monocular closure and were of normal size. It soon became obvious that 4C was still subdivided into left-eye and right-eye regions, as it is in normal animals, and that the cells in the stripes connected to the eye that had been closed were roughly normal. But the sequences of cells dominated by the closed eye were very brief, as if the stripes were abnormally narrow, around 0.2 millimeter instead of 0.4 or 0.5 millimeter. The stripes belonging to the open eye seemed correspondingly wider.

As soon as it became available, we used the anatomical technique of eye injection and transneuronal transport to obtain direct and vivid confirmation of this result. Following a few months' deprivation in a cat or monkey, we injected the good eye or the bad eye with radioactive amino acid. The autora-diographs showed a marked shrinkage of deprived-eye stripes and a corresponding expansion of the stripes belonging to the good eye. The lefthand photograph on this page shows the result of injecting the good eye with radioactive amino acid. The picture, taken, as usual, with dark-field illumination, shows a section cut parallel to the surface and passing through layer 4C. The narrow, pinched-off black stripes correspond to the eye that was closed: the wider light (labeled) stripes, to the open (injected) eye. The converse picture, in which the eye that had been closed was injected, is shown in the photograph on the next page. This section happens to be cut transverse to layer 4C, so we see the patches end-on.

These results in layer 4C tended to reinforce our doubts about the competition model, doubts that lingered on because of the geniculate-cell shrinkage:

Below: We obtained these sections from a macaque monkey that had an eye sutured closed from birth for eighteen months. The left (open) eye was then injected with radioactive amino acid, and after a week the brain was sectioned parallel to the surface of the visual cortex. (The cortex is dome shaped, so that cuts parallel to the surface are initially tangential, but then produce rings like onion rings, of progressively larger diameter. In the picture on the right, these have been cut from photographs and pasted together. We have since learned to flatten the cortex before freezing it, avoiding the cutting and pasting of serial sections.) In an ordinary photograph of a microscopic section the silver grains are black on a white background. Here we used dark-field microscopy, in which the silver grains scatter light and show as bright regions. The bright stripes, representing label in layer 4C from the open, injected eye, are widened, the dark ones (closed eye), are greatly narrowed.

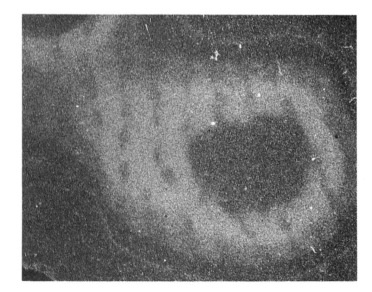

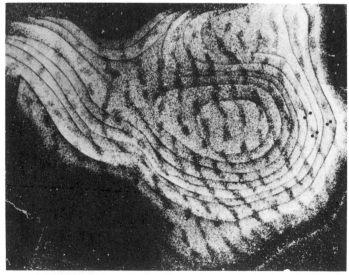

Here, in a different monkey, the closed eye
was injected. The section is transverse
rather than tangential. The stripes in layer
4C, seen end on and appearing bright in
this dark-field picture, are much shrunken.

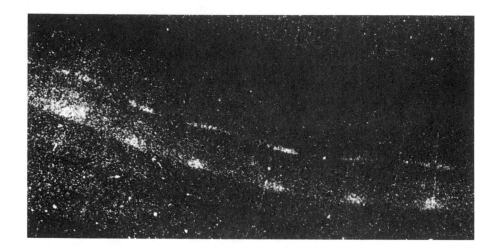

either the competition hypothesis was wrong or something was faulty somewhere in our reasoning. It turned out that the reasoning was at fault for both
the geniculate and the cortex. In the cortex, our mistake was in assuming that
when we closed the eyes in newborn animals, the ocular-dominance columns
were already well developed.

NORMAL DEVELOPMENT
OF EYE-DOMINANCE COLUMNS

The obvious way to learn about ocular-dominance columns in the
newborn was to check the distribution of fibers entering layer 4C by injecting
an eye on the first or second day of life. The result was surprising. Instead of
clear, crisp stripes, layer 4C showed a continuous smear of label. The lefthand
autoradiograph on the next page shows 4C cut transversely, and we see no
trace of columns. Only when we sliced the cortex parallel to its surface was it
possible to see a faint ripple at half-millimeter intervals, as shown in the right-
hand autoradiograph. Evidently, fibers from the geniculate that grow into the
cortex do not immediately go to and branch in separate left-eye and right-eye
regions. They first send branches everywhere over a radius of a few millimeters, and only later, around the time of birth, do they retract and adopt their
final distributions. The faint ripples in the newborn make it clear that the

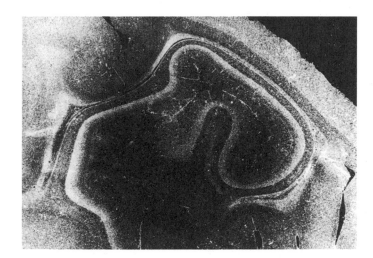 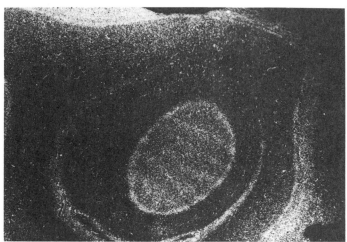

retraction has already begun before birth; in fact, by injecting the eyes of fetal monkeys (a difficult feat) Pasko Rakic has shown that it begins a few weeks before birth. By injecting one eye of monkeys at various ages after birth we could easily show that in the first two or three weeks a steady retraction of fiber terminals takes place in layer 4, so that by the fourth week the formation of the stripes is complete.

We easily confirmed the idea of postnatal retraction of terminals by making records from layer 4C in monkeys soon after birth. As the electrode traveled along the layer parallel to the surface, we could evoke activity from the two eyes at all points along the electrode track, instead of the crisp eye-alternation seen in adults. Carla Shatz has shown that an analogous process of development occurs in the cat geniculate: in fetal cats, many geniculate cells temporarily receive input from both eyes, but they lose one of the inputs as the layering becomes established.

The final pattern of left-eye, right-eye alternation in cortical layer 4C develops normally even if both eyes are sewn shut, indicating that the appropriate wiring can come about in the absence of experience. We suppose that during development, the incoming fibers from the two eyes compete in layer 4C in such a way that if one eye has the upper hand at any one place, the eye's advantage, in terms of numbers of nerve terminals, tends to increase, and the losing eye's terminals correspondingly recede. Any slight initial imbalance

Left: This section shows layer 4C cut transversely, from a newborn macaque monkey with an eye injected. The picture is dark field, so the radioactive label is bright. Its continuity shows that the terminals from each eye are not aggregated into stripes but are intermingled throughout the layer. (The white stripe between the exposed and buried 4C layers is white matter, full of fibers loaded with label on their way up from the lateral geniculates.) *Right:* Here the other hemisphere is cut so that the knife grazes the buried part of the striate cortex. We can now see hints of stripes in the upper part of 4C. (These stripes are in a subdivision related to the magnocellular geniculate layers. The deeper part, β, forms a continuous ring around α and so presumably is later in segregating.)

thus tends to increase progressively until, at age one month, the final punched-out stripes result, with complete domination everywhere in layer 4. In the case of eye closure, the balance is changed, and at the borders of the stripes, where normally the outcome would be a close battle, the open eye is favored and wins out, as shown in the diagram on this page.

We don't know what causes the initial imbalance during normal development, but in this unstable equilibrium presumably even the slightest difference would set things off. Why the pattern that develops should be one of parallel stripes, each a half-millimeter wide, is a matter of speculation. An idea several people espouse is that axons from the same eye attract each other over a short range but that left-eye and right-eye axons repel each other with a force that at short distances is weaker than the attracting forces, so that attraction wins. With increasing distance, the attracting force falls off more rapidly than the repelling force, so that farther away repulsion wins. The ranges of these competing tendencies determine the size of the columns. It seems from the mathematics that to get parallel stripes as opposed to a checkerboard or to islands of left-eye axons in a right-eye matrix, we need only specify that the boundaries between columns should be as short as possible.

One thus has a way of explaining the shrinkage and expansion of columns, by showing that at the time the eye was closed, early in life, competition was, after all, possible.

Ray Guillery, then at the University of Wisconsin, had meanwhile produced a plausible explanation for the atrophy of the geniculate cells. On examining our figures showing cell shrinkage in monocularly deprived cats, he noticed that in the part of the geniculate farthest out from the midline the shrinkage was much less; indeed, the cells there, in the temporal-crescent region, appeared to be normal. This region represents part of the visual field so far out to the side that only the eye on that side can see it, as shown in the diagram on

This competition model explains the segregation of fourth-layer fibers into eye-dominance columns. At birth the columns have already begun to form. Normally at any given point if one eye dominates even slightly, it ends up with a complete monopoly. If an eye is closed at birth, the fibers from the open eye still surviving at any given point in layer 4 take over completely. The only regions with persisting fibers from the closed eye are those where that eye had no competition when it was closed.

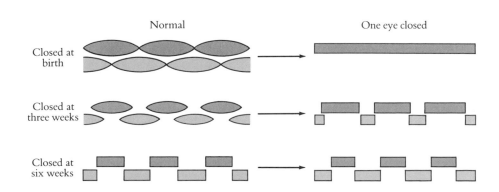

this page. We were distressed, to say the least; we had been so busy legitimizing our findings by measuring cell diameters that we had simply forgotten to look at our own pictures. This failure to atrophy of the cells in the geniculate receiving temporal-crescent projections suggested that the atrophy elsewhere in the geniculate might indeed be the result of competition and that out in the temporal crescent, where competition was absent, the deprived cells did not shrink.

By a most ingenious experiment, illustrated in the diagram on the next page, Murray Sherman and his colleagues went on to establish beyond any doubt the importance of competition in geniculate shrinkage. They first destroyed a tiny part of a kitten's retina in a region corresponding to an area of visual field that receives input from both eyes. Then they sutured closed the other eye. In the geniculate, severe cell atrophy was seen in a small area of the layer to which the eye with the local lesion projected. Many others had observed this result. The layer receiving input from the other eye, the one that had been closed, was also, as expected, generally shrunken, *except* in the area opposite the region of atrophy. There the cells were normal, despite the absence of visual input. By removing the competition, the atrophy from eye closure had been prevented. Clearly the competition could not be in the geniculate itself, but one has to remember that although the cell bodies and den-

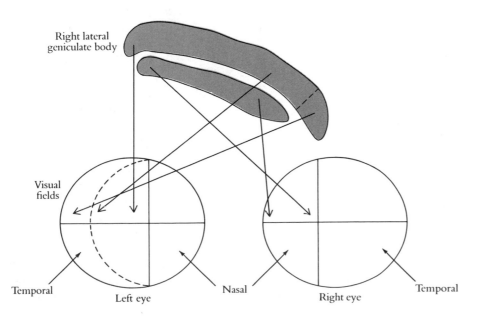

The various parts of the two retinas project onto their own areas of the right lateral geniculate body of the cat (seen in cross section). The upper geniculate layer, which receives input from the opposite (left) eye, overhangs the next layer. The overhanging part receives its input from the temporal crescent, the part of the contralateral nasal retina subserving the outer (temporal) part of the visual field, which has no counterpart in the other eye. (The temporal part of the visual field extends out farther because the nasal retina extends in farther). In monocular closure (here, for example, a closure of the left eye), the overhanging part doesn't atrophy, presumably because it has no competition from the right eye.

In 1974 an experiment by Sherman, Guillery, Kaas and Sanderson demonstrated the importance of competition in geniculate-cell shrinkage. If a small region of the left retina of a kitten is destroyed, there results an island of severe atrophy in the corresponding part of the upper layer of the right lateral geniculate body. If the right eye is then closed, the layer below the dorsal layer, as expected, becomes atrophic—except for the region immediately opposite the upper-layer atrophy, strongly suggesting a competitive origin for the atrophy resulting from eye closure.

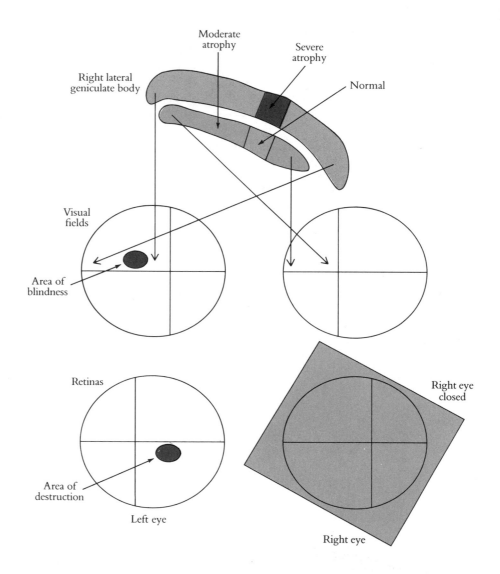

drites of the geniculate cells were in the geniculate, not all the cell was there: most of the axon terminals were in the cortex, and as I have described, the terminals belonging to a closed eye became badly shrunken. The conclusion is that in eye closures, the geniculate-cell shrinkage is a consequence of having fewer axon terminals to support.

The discovery that at birth layer 4 is occupied without interruption along its extent by fibers from both eyes was welcome because it explained how competition could occur at a synaptic level in a structure that had seemed to lack any opportunity for eye interaction. Yet the matter may not be quite as simple as this. If the reason for the changes in layer 4 was simply the opportunity for competition in the weeks after birth afforded by the mixture of eye inputs in that layer, then closing an eye at an age when the system is still plastic but the columns have separated should fail to produce the changes. We closed an eye at five-and-a-half weeks and injected the other eye after over a year of closure. The result was unequivocal shrinkage-expansion. This would seem to indicate that in addition to differential retraction of terminals, the result can be produced by sprouting of axon terminals into new territory.

FURTHER STUDIES
IN NEURAL PLASTICITY

The original experiments were followed by a host of others, carried out in many laboratories, investigating almost every imaginable kind of visual deprivation. One of the first and most interesting asked whether bringing up an animal so that it only saw stripes of one orientation would result in a loss of cells sensitive to all other orientations. In 1970 Colin Blakemore and G. F. Cooper, in Cambridge University, exposed kittens from an early age for a few hours each day to vertical black-and-white stripes but otherwise kept them in darkness. Cortical cells that preferred vertical orientation were preserved, but cells favoring other orientations declined dramatically in number. It is not clear whether cells originally having non-vertical orientations became unresponsive or whether they changed their preferences to vertical. Helmut Hirsch and Nico Spinelli, in a paper published the same year, employed goggles that let the cat see only vertical contours through one eye and only horizontal contours through the other. The result was a cortex containing cells that preferred verticals and cells that preferred horizontals, but few that preferred obliques. Moreover, cells activated by horizontal lines were influenced only by the eye exposed to the horizontal lines, and cells driven by vertical lines, only by the eye exposed to the vertical lines.

Other scientists have reared animals in a room that was dark except for a bright strobe light that flashed once or a few times every second; it showed the animal where it was but presumably minimized any perception of movement. The results of such experiments, done in 1975 by Max Cynader, Nancy Berman, and Alan Hein, at MIT, and by Max Cyander and G. Chernenko, at Dalhousie in Halifax, were all similar in producing a reduction of movement-selective cells. In another series of experiments by F. Tretter, Max Cynader, and Wolf Singer in Munich, animals were exposed to stripes moving from left to right; this led to the expected asymmetrical distribution of cortical direction-selective cells.

It seems natural to ask whether the physiological or anatomical changes produced by any of these deprivation experiments serve a useful purpose. If one eye is sewn closed at birth, does the expansion of the open eye's terrain in layer 4C confer any advantage on that eye? This question is still unanswered. It is hard to imagine that the acuity of the eye becomes better than normal, since ordinary acuity, the kind that the ophthalmologist measures with the test chart, ultimately depends on receptor spacing (Chapter 3), which is already at the limits imposed by the wavelength of light. In any case it seems most unlikely that such plasticity would have evolved just in case a baby lost an eye or developed strabismus. A more plausible idea is that the changes make use of a plasticity that evolved for some other function—perhaps for allowing the postnatal adjustments of connections necessary for form analysis, movement perception and stereopsis, where vision itself can act as a guide.

Although the deprivation experiments described in this chapter exposed animals to severely distorted environments, they have not involved direct assaults on the nervous system: no nerves were severed and no nervous tissue was destroyed. A number of recent studies have indicated that with more radical tampering even primary sensory areas can be rewired so as to produce gross rearrangements in topography. Moreover, the changes are not confined to a critical period in the early life of the animal, but can occur in the adult. Michael Merzenich at the University of California at San Francisco has shown that in the somatosensory system, after the nerves to a limb are severed or the limb amputated, the region of cortex previously supplied by these nerves ends up receiving input from neighboring areas of the body, for example from regions of skin bordering on the numb areas. A similar reorganization has been shown to occur in the visual system by Charles Gilbert and his colleagues at the Rockefeller University. They made small lesions in corresponding locations in the two retinas of a cat; when they later recorded from the area of striate cortex to which the damaged retinal areas had projected, they found that, far from being unresponsive, the cells responded actively to regions of retina adjacent to the damaged regions. In both these sets of experiments the cortical cells deprived of their normal sensory supply do not end up high and dry, but acquire new inputs. Their new receptive fields are much larger than normal, and thus by this measure the readjustments are crude. The changes seem to result in part from a heightening of the sensitivity of connections that had been present all along but had presumably been too weak to be easily detected, and in part from a subsequent, much slower development of new connections by a process known as nerve sprouting. Again it is not clear what such readjustments do for the animal; one would hardly expect to obtain a heightening of perception in the areas adjacent to numb or blind areas—indeed, given the large receptive fields, one would rather predict an impairment.

THE ROLE OF PATTERNED ACTIVITY IN NEURAL DEVELOPMENT

Over the past few years a set of most impressive advances have forced an entire rethinking of the mechanisms responsible for the laying down of neural connections, both before and after birth. The discovery of orientation selectivity and orientation columns in newborn monkeys had seemed to indicate a strongly genetic basis for the detailed cortical wiring. Yet it seemed unlikely that the genome could contain enough information to account for all that specificity. After birth, to be sure, the visual cortex could fine-tune its neural connections in response to the exigencies of the environment, but it was hard to imagine how any such environmental molding could account for prenatal wiring.

Our outlook has been radically changed by a heightened appreciation of the part played in development by neural activity. The strabismus experiments had pointed to the importance of the relative timing of impulses arriving at the cortex, but the first direct evidence that firing was essential to the formation of neural connections came from experiments by Michael Stryker and William Harris at Harvard Medical School in 1986. They managed to eliminate impulse activity in the optic nerves by repeatedly injecting tetrodotoxin (a neurotoxin obtained from the puffer fish) into the eyes of kittens, over a period beginning at age 2 weeks and extending to an age of 6 to 8 weeks. Then the injections were discontinued and activity was allowed to resume. By the eighth week after birth the ocular dominance columns in cats normally show clear signs of segregation, but microelectrode recordings indicated that the temporary impulse blockade had prevented the segregation completely. Clearly, then, the segregation must depend on impulses coming into the cortex.

In another set of experiments Stryker and S. L. Strickland asked if it was important for the activity of impulses in optic-nerve fibers to be synchronized, within each eye and between the two eyes. They again blocked optic-nerve impulses in the eyes with tetrodotoxin, but this time they electrically stimulated the optic nerves during the entire period of blockage. In one set of kittens they stimulated both optic nerves together and in this way artificially synchronized inputs both within each eye and between the eyes. In these animals the recordings again indicated that the formation of ocular dominance columns had been completely blocked. In a second set of kittens they stimulated the two nerves alternately, shocking one nerve for 8 seconds, then the other. In this case the columns showed an exaggerated segregation similar to that obtained with artificial strabismus. The normal partial segregation of ocular dominance columns may thus be regarded as the result of two competing processes: in the first, segregation is promoted when neural activity is synchronized in each eye but not correlated between the eyes; and in the second, binocular innervation of neurons and merging of the two sets of columns is promoted by the synchrony between corresponding retinal areas of the two eyes that results from normal binocular vision.

Carla Shatz and her colleagues have discovered that a similar process occurs prior to birth in the lateral geniculate body. In the embryo the two optic nerves grow into the geniculate and initially spread out to occupy all the layers. At this stage many cells receive inputs from both eyes. Subsequently segregation begins, and by a few weeks before birth the two sets of nerve terminals have become confined to their proper layers. The segregation seems to depend on spontaneous activity, which has been shown by Lamberto Maffei and L. Galli-Resta to be present in fetal optic nerves, even before the rods and cones have developed. Shatz and her colleagues showed that if this normal spontaneous firing is suppressed by injecting tetrodotoxin into the eyes of the embryo, the segregation into layers is prevented.

Further evidence for the potential importance of synchrony in development of neuronal connections comes from work at Stanford by Dennis Baylor, Rachel Wong, Marcus Meister, and Carla Shatz. They used a new technique for recording simultaneously from up to one hundred retinal ganglion cells. They found that the spontaneous firing of ganglion cells in fetal retinas tends to begin at some focus in the retina and to spread across in a wave. Each wave lasts several seconds and successive waves occur at intervals of up to a minute or so, starting at random from different locations and proceeding in random directions. The result is a strong tendency for neighboring cells to fire in synchrony, but almost certainly no tendency for cells in corresponding local areas of the two retinas to fire in synchrony. They suggest that this local retinal synchrony, plus the lack of synchrony between the two eyes, may form the basis for the layering in the lateral geniculate, the ocular dominance columns in the cortex, and the detailed topographic maps in both structures. Shatz has summed up the idea by the slogan "Cells that fire together wire together".

This concept could explain why, as discussed in Chapter 5, nerve cells with like response properties tend to be grouped together. There the topic was the aggregation of cells with like orientation selectivities into orientation columns, and I stressed the advantages of such aggregation for economy in lengths of connections. Now we see that it may be the synchronous firing of the cells that promotes the grouping. How, then, do we account for the fact that connections responsible for orientation selectivity are already present at birth, without benefit of prior retinal stimulation by contours? Can we avoid the conclusion that these connections, at least, must be genetically determined? It seems to me that one highly speculative possibility is offered by the waves of activity that criss-cross the fetal retina: if each wave spreads out from a focus, a different focus each time, perhaps the advancing fronts of the waves supply just the oriented stimuli that are required to achieve the appropriate synchrony—an oriented moving line. One could even imagine testing such an idea by stimulating the fetal retina to produce waves that always spread out from the same focus, to see if that would lead to all cortical cells having the same orientation selectivity.

All of this reinforces the idea that activity is important if competition is to take place. This is true for the competition between the two eyes that occurs in normal development, and the abnormal competition that occurs in deprivation and strabismus. Beyond that, it is not just the presence or absence of activity that counts, but rather the patterns of synchronization of the activity.

THE BROADER IMPLICATIONS OF DEPRIVATION RESULTS

The deprivation experiments described in this chapter have shown that it is possible to produce tangible physiological and structural changes in the nervous system by distorting an animal's experience. As already emphasized, none of the procedures did direct damage to the nervous system; instead the trauma was environmental, and in each case, the punishment has more or less fit the crime. Exclude form, and cells whose normal responses are to forms become unresponsive to them. Unbalance the eyes by cutting a muscle, and the connections that normally subserve binocular interactions become disrupted. Exclude movement, or movement in some particular direction, and the cells that would have responded to these movements no longer do so.

It hardly requires a leap of the imagination to ask whether a child deprived of social contacts—left in bed all day to gaze at an orphanage ceiling—or an animal raised in isolation, as in some of Harry Harlow's experiments, may not suffer analogous, equally palpable changes in some brain region concerned with relating to other animals of the same species. To be sure, no pathologist has yet seen such changes, but even in the visually deprived cortex, without very special methods such as axon-transport labels or deoxyglucose, no changes can be seen either. When some axons retract, others advance, and the structure viewed even with an electron microscope continues to look perfectly normal. Conceivably, then, many conditions previously categorized by psychiatrists as "functional" may turn out to involve organic defects. And perhaps treatments such as psychotherapy may be a means of gaining access to these higher brain regions, just as one tries in cases of strabismic amblyopia to gain access to the striate cortex by specific forms of binocular eye stimulation.

Our notions of the possible implications of this type of work thus go far beyond the visual system—into neurology and much of psychiatry. Freud could have been right in attributing psychoneuroses to abnormal experiences in childhood, and considering that his training was in neurology, my guess is that he would have been delighted at the idea that such childhood experiences might produce tangible histological or histochemical changes in the real, physical brain.

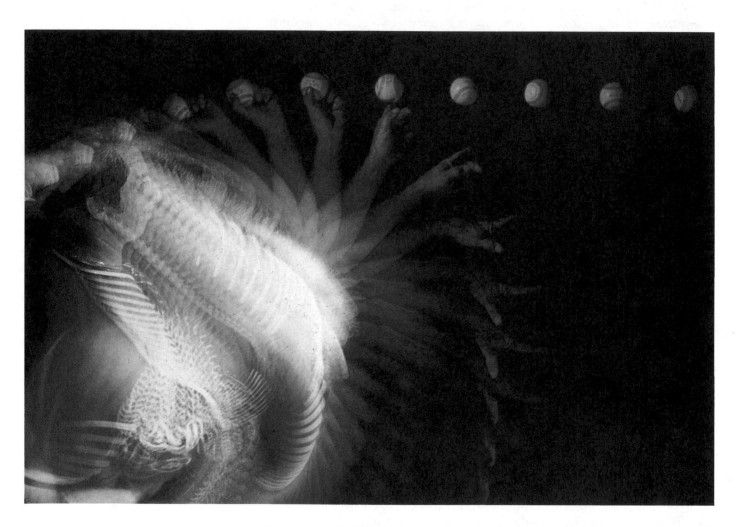

To throw a strike, a pitcher must project the ball over a plate about 1 foot wide, 60.5 feet away—a target that subtends an angle of about 1 degree, about twice the apparent size of the moon. To accomplish such a feat, with velocity and spin, requires excellent vision plus the ability to regulate the force and timing of over a hundred muscles. A batter to connect with the ball must judge its exact position less than a second after its release. The success or failure of either feat depends on visual circuits—all those discussed in this book and many at higher visual levels—and motor circuits involving motor cortex, cerebellum, brainstem, and spinal cord.

10

PRESENT AND FUTURE

My intention in writing this book was to describe what we know of the anatomy and physiology of the visual pathway up to the striate cortex. The knowledge we have now is really only the beginning of an effort to understand the physiological basis of perception, a story whose next stages are just coming into view; we can see major mountain ranges in the middle distance, but the end is nowhere in sight.

The striate cortex is just the first of over a dozen separate visual areas, each of which maps the whole visual field. These areas collectively form the patchwork quilt that constitutes the occipital cortex and extends forward into the posterior temporal cortex and posterior parietal cortex. Beginning with the striate cortex, each area feeds into two or more areas higher in the hierarchy, and the connections are topographically organized so that any given area contains an orderly representation of the visual field, just as the striate cortex does. The ascending connections presumably take the visual information from one region to the next for further processing. For each of these areas our problem is to find out how the information is processed—the same problem we faced earlier when we asked what the striate cortex does with the information it gets from the geniculate.

Although we have only recently come to realize how numerous these visual areas are, we are already building up knowledge about the connections and single-cell physiology of some of them. Just as area 17 is a mosaic of two sets of regions, blob and nonblob, so the next visual area, area 18 or visual area 2, is a mosaic of three sets. Unlike the blobs and interblobs, which formed islands in an ocean, the mosaic in area 18 takes the form of parallel stripes. In these subdivisions we find a striking segregation of function. In the set of thick stripes, most of the cells are highly sensitive to the relative horizontal positions of the stimuli in the two eyes, as described in Chapter 7; we therefore conclude that this thick-stripe subdivision is concerned at least in part with stereopsis. In the second set, the thin stripes, cells lack orientation selectivity and often show specific color responses. In the third set, the pale stripes, cells are orientation selective and most are end stopped. Thus the three sets of subdivisions that make up area 18 seem to be concerned with stereopsis, color, and form.

A similar division of labor occurs in the areas beyond area 18, but now entire areas seem to be given over to one or perhaps two visual functions. An area called MT (for middle temporal gyrus) is devoted to movement and stereopsis; one called V 4 (V for visual) seems to be concerned mainly with color. We can thus discern two processes that go hand in hand. The first is hierarchical. To solve the various problems in vision outlined in previous chapters—color, stereopsis, movement, form—information is operated upon in one area after the next, with progressive abstraction and increasing complexity of representation. The second process consists of a divergence of pathways. Apparently the problems require such different strategies and hardware that it becomes more efficient to handle them in entirely separate channels.

This surprising tendency for attributes such as form, color, and movement to be handled by separate structures in the brain immediately raises the question of how all the information is finally assembled, say for perceiving a bouncing red ball. It obviously must be assembled somewhere, if only at the motor nerves that subserve the action of catching. Where it's assembled, and how, we have no idea.

This is where we are, in 1995, in the step-by-step analysis of the visual path. In terms of numbers of synapses (perhaps eight or ten) and complexity of transformations, it may seem a long way from the rods and cones in the retina to areas MT or visual area 2 in the cortex, but it is surely a far longer way from such processes as orientation tuning, end-stopping, disparity tuning, or color opponency to the recognition of any of the shapes that we perceive in our everyday life. We are far from understanding the perception of objects, even such comparatively simple ones as a circle, a triangle, or the letter A—indeed, we are far from even being able to come up with plausible hypotheses.

We should not be particularly surprised or disconcerted over our relative ignorance in the face of such mysteries. Those who work in the field of artificial intelligence (AI) cannot design a machine that begins to rival the brain at carrying out such special tasks as processing the written word, driving a car along a road, or distinguishing faces. They have, however, shown that the theoretical difficulties in accomplishing any of these tasks are formidable. It is not that the difficulties cannot be solved—the brain clearly has solved them— but rather that the methods the brain applies cannot be simple: in the lingo of AI, the problems are "nontrivial". So the brain solves nontrivial problems. The remarkable thing is that it solves not just two or three but thousands of them.

In the question period following a lecture, a sensory physiologist or psychologist soon gets used to being asked what the best guess is as to how objects are recognized. Do cells continue to become more and more specialized at more and more central levels, so that at some stage we can expect to find cells so specialized that they respond to one single person's face—say, one's grandmother's? This notion, called the *grandmother cell theory,* is hard to entertain seriously. Would we expect to find separate cells for grandmother smiling, grandmother weeping, or grandmother sewing? Separate cells for the concept or definition of grandmother: one's mother's or father's mother? And if we did have grandmother cells, then what? Where would they project?

The alternative is to suppose that a given object leads to the firing of a particular constellation of cells, any member of which could also belong to other constellations. Knowing as we do that destroying a small region of brain does not generally destroy specific memories, we have to suppose that the cells in a constellation are not localized to a single cortical area, but extend over many areas. Grandmother sewing then becomes a bigger constellation comprising grandmother-by-definition, grandmother's face, and sewing.

It is admittedly not easy to think of a way to get at such ideas experimentally. To record from one cell alone and make sense of the results even in the striate cortex is not easy: it is hard even to imagine coming to terms with a cell that may be a member of a hundred constellations, each consisting of a thousand cells. Having tried to record from three cells simultaneously and understand what they all are doing in the animal's daily life, I can only admire the efforts of those who hope to build electrode arrays to record simultaneously from hundreds. But by now we should be used to seeing problems solved that only yesterday seemed insuperable.

Running counter to wooly ideas about constellations of cells is long-standing and still accumulating evidence for the existence of cortical regions specialized for face perception. Charles Gross's group at Princeton has recorded from cells in the monkey, in a visual area of the temporal lobe, that seem to respond selectively to faces. And humans with strokes in one particular part of the inferior occipital lobe often lose the ability to recognize faces, even those of close relatives. Antonio Damasio, at the University of Iowa, has suggested that these patients have lost the ability to distinguish not just faces but a broader class of objects that includes faces. He describes a woman who could recognize neither faces nor individual cars. She could tell a car from a truck, but to find her own car in a parking lot she had to walk along reading off the license plate numbers, which suggests that her vision and her ability to read numbers were both intact.

Speculating can be fun, but when can we hope to have answers to some of these questions about perception? Some thirty-seven years have passed since Kuffler worked out the properties of retinal ganglion cells. In the interval the way we view both the complexity of the visual pathway and the range of problems posed by perception has radically changed. We realize that discoveries such as center-surround receptive fields and orientation selectivity represent merely two steps in unraveling a puzzle that contains hundreds of such steps. The brain has many tasks to perform, even in vision, and millions of years of evolution have produced solutions of great ingenuity. With hard work we may come to understand any small subset of these, but it seems unlikely that we will be able to tackle them all. It would be just as unrealistic to suppose that we could ever understand the intricate workings of each of the millions of proteins floating around in our bodies. Philosophically, however, it is important to have at least a few examples—of neural circuits or proteins—that we do understand well: our ability to unravel even a few of the processes responsible for life—or for perception, thought, or emotions—tells us that total understanding is *in principle* possible, that we do not need to appeal to mystical life forces—or to the mind.

Some may fear that such a materialistic outlook, which regards the brain as a kind of super machine, will take the magic out of life and deprive us of all spiritual values. This is about the same as fearing that a knowledge of human anatomy will prevent us from admiring the human form. Art students and medical students know that the opposite is true. The problem is with the words: if *machine* implies something with rivets and ratchets and gears, that does sound unromantic. But by *machine* I mean any object that does tasks in a way that is consonant with the laws of physics, an object that we can ultimately understand in the same way we understand a printing press. I believe the brain is such an object.

Do we need to worry about possible dire consequences of understanding the brain, analogous to the consequences of understanding the atom? Do we have to worry about the CIA reading or controlling our thoughts? I see no cause for loss of sleep, at least not for the next century or so. It should be obvious from all the preceding chapters of this book that reading or directing thoughts by neurophysiological means is about as feasible as a weekend trip to the Andromeda galaxy and back. But even if thought control turns out to be possible in principle, the prevention or cure of millions of schizophrenics should be easy by comparison. I would prefer to take the gamble, and continue to do research.

We may soon have to face a different kind of problem: that of reconciling some of our most cherished and deep-seated beliefs with new knowledge of the brain. In 1983, the Church of Rome formally indicated its acceptance of the physics and cosmology Gallileo had promulgated 350 years earlier. Today our courts, politicians, and publishers are struggling with the same problem in teaching school children the facts about evolution and molecular biology. If mind and soul are to neurobiology what sky and heaven are to astronomy and The Creation is to biology, then a third revolution in thought may be in the offing. We should not, however, smugly regard these as struggles between scientific wisdom and religious ignorance. If humans tend to cherish certain beliefs, it is only reasonable to suppose that our brains have evolved so as to favor that tendency—for reasons concerned with survival. To dismantle old beliefs or myths and replace them with scientific modes of thought should not and probably cannot be done hastily or by decree. But it seems to me that we will, in the end, have to modify our beliefs to make room for facts that our brains have enabled us to establish by experiment and deduction: the world is round; it goes around the sun; living things evolve; life can be explained in terms of fantastically complex molecules; and thought may some day be explained in terms of fantastically complex sets of neural connections.

The potential gains in understanding the brain include more than the cure and prevention of neurologic and psychiatric diseases. They go well beyond that, to fields like education. In educating, we are trying to influence the brain: how could we fail to teach better, if we understood the thing we are trying to influence? Possible gains extend even to art, music, athletics, and social relationships. Everything we do depends on our brains.

Having said all this, I must admit that what most strongly motivates me, and I think most of my colleagues, is sheer curiosity over the workings of the most complicated structure known.

FURTHER READING

Chapter 1

Scientific American issue on the brain, 241(3), September 1979. Reprinted as *The Brain, A Scientific American Book,* W. H. Freeman, New York, 1979.

Nauta, W. J. H., and M. Feirtag: *Fundamental Neuroanatomy,* W. H. Freeman, New York, 1986.

Ramón y Cajal, Santiago: *Histologie du Système Nerveux de l'Homme et des Vertébrés,* vols. 1 and 2 (translated by L. Azoulay from the Spanish), Madrid, 1952.

Chapter 2

Kandel, E. R., J. H. Schwartz, and T. M. Jessell: *Principles of Neural Science,* 3d ed., Elsevier North-Holland, New York, 1991.

Nicholls, J. G., A. R. Martin, and B. G. Wallace: *From Neuron to Brain,* 3d ed., Sinauer Associates, Sunderland, Mass., 1992.

Chapter 3

Dowling, J. E.: *The Retina—An Approachable Part of the Brain,* Harvard University Press, Cambridge, Mass., 1987.

Kuffler, S. W.: Neurons in the retina: Organization, inhibition and excitatory problems. *Cold Spring Harbor Symposia on Quantitative Biology* 17: 281–292 (1952).

Nicholls, J. G., A. R. Martin, and B. G. Wallace: *From Neuron to Brain,* 3d ed., Sinauer Associates, Sunderland, Mass., 1992.

Schnapf, J. L., and D. A. Baylor: How photoreceptor cells respond to light. *Sci. Am.* 256: 40–47 (1987).

Chapter 4

Hubel, D. H., and T. N. Wiesel: Receptive fields of single neurones in the cat's striate cortex. *J. Physiol.* 148: 574–591 (1959).

—— and ——: Receptive fields, binocular interaction and functional architecture in the cat's visual cortex. *J. Physiol.* 160: 106–154 (1962).

—— and ——: Receptive fields and functional architecture in two non-striate visual areas (18 and 19) of the cat. *J. Neurophysiol.* 28: 229–289 (1965).

—— and ——: Receptive fields and functional architecture of monkey striate cortex. *J. Physiology.* 195: 215–243 (1968).

—— and ——: Brain mechanisms of vision. *Sci. Am.* 241: 130–144 (1979).

Hubel, D. H.: Exploration of the primary visual cortex, 1955–78 (Nobel Lecture). *Nature* 299: 515–524 (1982).

Chapters 5 and 6

Hubel, D. H., and T. N. Wiesel: Functional architecture of macaque monkey visual cortex (Ferrier Lecture). *Proc. R. Soc. Lond.* B 198: 1–59 (1977).

Hubel, D. H.: Exploration of the primary visual cortex, 1955–78 (Nobel Lecture). *Nature* 299: 515–524 (1982).

Chapter 7

Sperry, Roger: "Some effects of disconnecting the cerebral hemispheres" (Nobel Lecture, 8 Dec. 1981), in *Les Prix Nobel,* Almqvist & Wiksell International, Stockholm, 1982.

Gazzaniga, M. S., J. E. Bogen, and R. W. Sperry: Observations on visual perception after disconnexion of the cerebral hemispheres in man. *Brain* 88: 221–236 (1965).

Gazzaniga, M. S., and R. W. Sperry: Language after section of the cerebral commissures. *Brain* 90: 131–148 (1967).

Lepore, F., M. Ptito, and H. H. Jasper: *Two Hemispheres—One Brain: Functions of the Corpus Callosum,* Alan R. Liss, New York, 1984.

Julesz, Bela: *Foundations of Cyclopean Perception,* University of Chicago Press, Chicago, 1971.

Poggio, G. F., and B. Fischer: Binocular interaction and depth sensitivity of striate and prestriate cortical neurons of the behaving rhesus monkey. *J. Neurophysiol.* 40: 1392–1405 (1977).

Chapter 8

Daw, N. W.: The psychology and physiology of colour vision. *Trends in Neurosci.* 7: 330–335 (1984).

Hering, Ewald: *Outlines of a Theory of the Light Sense* (translated by Leo M. Hurvich and Dorothea Jameson), Harvard University Press, Cambridge, Mass., 1964.

Ingle, D.: The goldfish as a Retinex animal. *Science* 227: 651–654 (1985).

Land, E. H.: An alternative technique for the computation of the designator in the Retinex theory of color vision. *Proc. Natl. Acad. Sci. USA* 83: 3078–3080 (1986).

Livingstone, M. S., and D. H. Hubel: Anatomy and physiology of a color system in the primate visual cortex. *J. Neurosci.* 4: 309–356 (1984).

Nathans, J.: Genes for color vision. *Sci. Am.* 260: 42–49 (1989).

Schnapf, J. L., and D. A. Baylor: How photoreceptor cells respond to light. *Sci. Am.* 256: 40–47 (1987).

Southall, J. P. C. (ed.): *Helmholtz's Treatise on Physiological Optics* (translated from 3d German edition), 3 vols. bound as 2, Dover Publishers, New York, 1962.

Chapter 9

Hubel, D. H.: Effects of deprivation on the visual cortex of cat and monkey, *Harvey Lectures,* Series 72, Academic Press, New York, 1978, pp. 1–51.

Wiesel, T. N.: Postnatal development of the visual cortex and the influence of environment (Nobel Lecture). *Nature* 299: 583–591 (1982).

Wiesel, T. N., and Hubel, D. H.: Effects of visual deprivation on morphology and physiology of cells in the cat's lateral geniculate body. *J. Neurophysiol.* 26: 978–993 (1963).

—— and ——: Receptive fields of cells in striate cortex of very young, visually inexperienced kittens. *J. Neurophysiol.* 26: 994–1002 (1963).

—— and ——: Single-cell responses in striate cortex of kittens deprived of vision in one eye. *J. Neurophysiol.* 26: 1003–1017 (1963).

—— and ——: Comparison of the effects of unilateral and bilateral eye closure on cortical unit responses in kittens. *J. Neurophysiol.* 28: 1029–1040 (1965).

—— and ——: Binocular interaction in striate cortex of kittens reared with artificial squint. *J. Neurophysiol.* 28: 1041–1059 (1965).

—— and ——: Extent of recovery from the effects of visual deprivation in kittens. *J. Neurophysiol.* 28: 1060–1072 (1965).

Hubel, D. H., T. N. Wiesel, and S. LeVay: Plasticity of ocular dominance columns in monkey striate cortex. *Phil. Trans. R. Soc. Lond. B,* 278: 377–409 (1977).

Shatz, C. J.: The developing brain. *Sci. Am.* 267: 60–67 (1992).

Chapter 10

Crick, F. H. C.: Thinking about the brain. *Sci. Am.* 241: 219–233 (1979).

Hubel, D. H.: "Neurobiology: A science in need of a Copernicus," in J. Neyman (ed.), *The Heritage of Copernicus,* Part II, M.I.T. Press, Cambridge, Mass., pp. 243–260.

Van Essen, D. C., and J. H. R. Maunsell: Hierarchical organization and functional streams in the visual cortex. *Trends in Neurosci.* 6: 370–375 (1983).

SOURCES OF ILLUSTRATIONS

Illustrations by
Carol Donner
Tom Cardamone Associates

Frontispiece
Joseph Gagliardi

Facing page 1
Cajal Institute

Page 3
by Carol Donner

Page 5
Art by Carol Donner

Page 6 (left, middle), page 7
Drawings by Santiago Ramón y Cajal.
From *Histologie du Système Nerveux de l'Homme et des Vertébrés,* Madrid, 1952.

Page 6 (right)
Jennifer Lund, *J. Comp. Neurology* 257: 60–92 (1987).

Page 9
Art by Carol Donner

Page 12
Drawing by Santiago Ramón y Cajal.
Painted by R. Padró.

Page 15
Sanford L. Palay, Harvard Medical School

Page 19
Cedric Raine, Albert Einstein College of Medicine

Page 23
Barbara Reese, National Institutes of Health

Page 30
Art by Carol Donner

Page 34
Art by Carol Donner

Page 35
© Lennart Nilsson. From his book *Behold Man,* Little, Brown, and Company, Boston.

Page 38
Artwork by Carol Donner

Page 40
Janet Robbins, Harvard Medical School

Page 48
Elio Raviola, Harvard Medical School

Page 48
S. Polyak. From *The Retina,* University of Chicago Press, Chicago, 1941.

Page 50
Akimichi Kaneko

Page 58
Fritz Goro

Page 60
Artwork by Carol Donner

Page 62
David H. Hubel

Page 65
David H. Hubel

Page 68
Janet Robbins, Harvard Medical School

Page 70
Adapted from David H. Hubel. *J. Physiol.* 148: 574–591 (1959), Fig. 8.

Page 74
Adapted from David H. Hubel and Torsten N. Wiesel, *J. Physiol.* 160: 106–154 (1962), Fig. 19.

Page 75 (top)
James P. Kelly, Columbia University

Pages 75 (bottom), 76, and 77
Adapted from David H. Hubel and Torsten N. Wiesel, *J. Physiol.* 160: 106–154 (1962), Figs. 7, 20, and 8.

Page 80
From A. L. Yarbus, *Eye Movements and Vision,* Plenum, New York, 1967.

Page 89 (left)
From David H. Hubel and Torsten N. Wiesel, *J. Physiol.* 160: 106–154 (1962), Fig. 17.

Page 89 (right)
From David H. Hubel, *Harvey Lectures,* series 72, Academic Press, New York, 1978, Fig. 6.

Page 90
From David H. Hubel and Torsten N. Wiesel, *J. Physiol.* 160: 106–154 (1962), Fig. 10

Page 92
From David H. Hubel and Torsten N. Wiesel, Ferrier Lecture, *Proc. R. Soc.* 198: 1–59.

Page 94
Montreal Neurological Institute

Pages 95, 96, and 97
From David H. Hubel and Torsten N.
Wiesel, Ferrier Lecture, *Proc. R. Soc.*
198: 1–59, Figs. 6a, 6b, and 10.

Page 98
Drawing by Santiago Ramón y Cajal.

Pages 109, 110, and 111
From David H. Hubel and Torsten N.
Wiesel, Ferrier Lecture, *Proc. R. Soc.*
198: 1–59, Figs. 21, 22, and 23.

Page 112 (bottom)
From Simon LeVay, David H. Hubel,
and Torsten N. Wiesel, *J. Comp.
Neurol.* 159: 559–576.

Page 113
Adapted from C. Kennedy et al., *Proceedings of the National Academy of Sciences* 73: 4230–4234 (1976), Fig. 2.

Page 114
From Roger Tootell et al., Deoxyglucose Analysis of Retinotopic Organization in Primate Streate Cortex, *Science* 218: 902–904 (1982), Fig. 1.

Pages 116 and 117
From David H. Hubel and Torsten N.
Wiesel, *J. Comp. Neurol.* 158: 267–294, Fig. 1.

Page 118
From David H. Hubel and Torsten N.
Wiesel, *J. Physiol.* 195: 215–243 (1968), Fig. 9.

Page 119 (top)
From David H. Hubel and Torsten N.
Wiesel, *J. Comp. Neurol.* 158: 267–294 (1974), Fig. 8c.

Page 121 (top and bottom)
From David H. Hubel, Torsten N.
Wiesel, and M. P. Stryker, *J. Comp.
Neurol.* 177: 361–379 (1978), Fig. 7c.

Page 122
Gary Blasdel, University of Calgary

Page 124
From David H. Hubel and Torsten N.
Wiesel, Ferrier Lecture, *Proc. R. Soc.*
198: 1–59 (1977), Fig. 28.

Page 128
Janet Robbins, Harvard Medical
School

Pages 128 and 129 (top)
From David H. Hubel and Torsten N.
Wiesel, Uniformity of Monkey Striate
Cortex: A Parallel Relationship between Field Size, Scatter, and Magnification Factor, *J. Comp. Neurol.* 158: 295–306 (1974), Figs. 1 and 2.

Page 129
From David H. Hubel, Nobel Lecture, *Nature* 299: 515–524 (1982), Fig. 14.

Page 133
From David H. Hubel and Torsten N.
Wiesel, Ferrier Lecture, *Proc. R. Soc.*
198: 1–59 (1977), Fig. 14.

Page 134
Adapted from P. M. Daniel and
David Whitteridge, *J. Physiol.* 159: 203–221 (1961), Fig. 6.

Page 136
David H. Hubel

Pages 138 and 139
Art by Carol Donner

Page 142
From David H. Hubel and Torsten N.
Wiesel, *J. Neurophysiol.* 30: 1561–1573 (1967), Fig. 4.

Page 148 (left)
ET Archive Ltd.

Page 148 (right)
Sir Charles Wheatstone, Contribution
to the Physiology of Vision, *Phil.
Trans. R. Soc.* (1838).

Page 150
From Bela Julesz, *Foundations of Cyclopean Perception*, University of Chicago Press, Chicago and London, 1971, p. 319.

Pages 152 and 153
From Margaret S. Livingstone and
David H. Hubel, *J. Neurosci.*, in press.

Page 158
Charles Arneson

Page 169
Nancy Rodger

Page 176
Edwin Land

Page 177
Photo from Edwin Land. From D. J.
Ingle, The Goldfish as a Retinex Animal, *Science* 227: 651–653 (1985).

Page 179
From Gunnar Svaetichin and Edward
F. MacNichol, Jr., *Annals of the New
York Academy of Sciences,* 74: 385–404 (1958).

Pages 184 and 185
From Margaret S. Livingstone and
David H. Hubel, Anatomy and Physiology of a Color System in the Primate Visual Cortex, *J. Neurosci.* 4: 309–356 (1984), Figs. 32 and 31.

Page 190
Chip Clark

Page 194 (top left)
From Torsten N. Wiesel and David
H. Hubel, *J. of Neurophysiol.* 26: 1003–1017 (1963), Fig. 3.

Page 194 (top right)
From David H. Hubel and Torsten N.
Wiesel, *J. of Physiol.* 160: 106–154 (1962), Fig. 12.

Page 194 (bottom left)
From David H. Hubel, Torsten N.
Wiesel, and Simon LeVay, *Phil. Trans.* 278: 377–409 (1977), Fig. 1.

Page 194 (bottom right)
From David H. Hubel, *Harvey Lectures,* series 73, Academic Press, 1978, Fig. 6.

Page 196
From Torsten N. Wiesel and David H. Hubel, *J. of Neurophysiol.* 26: 978–993 (1963), Fig. 1.

Page 199 (left)
From Torsten N. Wiesel, Nobel Lecture, *Nature* 299: 583–591 (1982), Fig. 2.

Page 199 (middle)
From David H. Hubel, *Harvey Lecture,* series 72, Academic Press, 1978, Fig. 18.

Page 200 (left and right)
From David H. Hubel, *Harvey Lecture,* series 72, Academic Press, 1978, Figs. 19 and 20.

Page 201
Francois Gohier/Ardea, London

Page 202 (top)
June E. Armstrong/New England Regional Primate Research Center

Page 202 (bottom)
From Torsten N. Wiesel and David H. Hubel, *J. Comp. Neurol.* 158: 307–318 (1974), Fig. 2.

Page 206
From David H. Hubel and Torsten N. Wiesel, *J. Neurophysiol.* 28: 1041–1059 (1965), Fig. 5.

Pages 209, 210, 211, and 212
From David H. Hubel, Torsten N. Wiesel, and Simon LeVay, *Phil. Trans. R. Soc.* 278: 377–409 (1977), Figs. 15, 22, 25, and 28.

Page 218
Gordon Gahan

INDEX

Page numbers in *italics* refer to illustrations.
Page numbers in **boldface** refer to the main discussion of a topic.

Selected hardcover books in the Scientific American Library Series

Other Scientific American Library books now available in paperback

If you would like to purchase additional volumes in the Scientific American Library, please send your order to:

Scientific American Library
P. O. Box 646
Holmes, PA 19043-9946